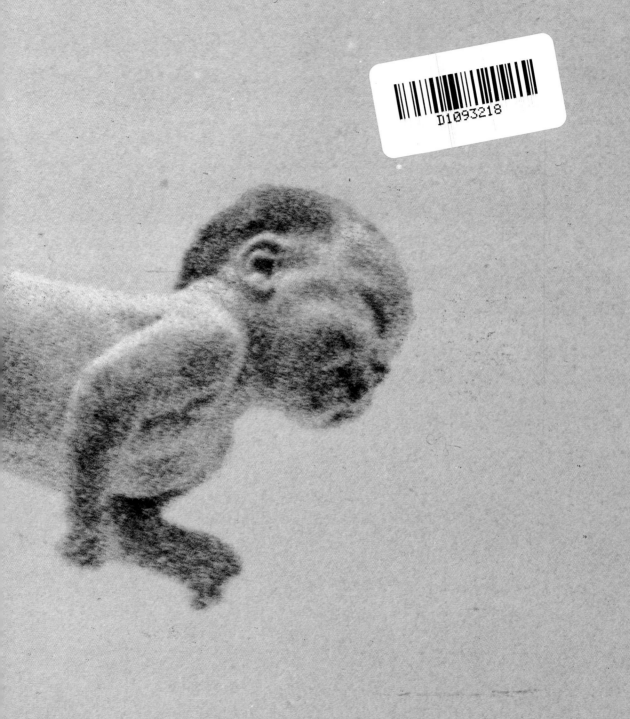

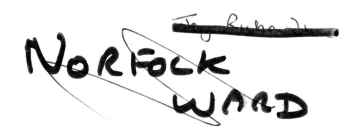

Norfolk
 WARD

WATER BABIES

ERIK SIDENBLADH
WATER

BABIES

Igor Tjarkovsky and
his methods of delivering
and training children in water

Adam & Charles Black · London

This edition first published 1983
A & C Black (Publishers) Ltd
35 Bedford Row, London WC1R 4JH

ISBN 0-7136-2319-5

Originally published by Akademilitteratur AB
Stockholm, with the title Vattenbarn

© 1982 (text) Erik Sidenbladh and Akademilitteratur AB
© 1982 (photographs) Akademilitteratur AB

English translation by Wendy Croton

Filmset by August Filmsetting, Warrington, Cheshire

Printed by L.E.G.O. S.p.A. in Vicenza, Italy

Contents

Preface

Water Babies is about a constructive new approach to childbirth and child-rearing, developed by the Soviet researcher, Igor Tjarkovsky.

At a time when most routes towards constructive changes in human life seem either blocked or frightening, we felt it was important to publish this book. It describes how one man's vision and determination can open up new avenues leading to a better and fuller life for human beings.

Igor Tjarkovsky, like all visionaries, carries his work far beyond respect for dogma and generally accepted ideas. Many of the ideas in this book may be new to the Western public. Tjarkovsky makes statements which conflict with the ideas of our scientific establishment. Tjarkovsky is Russian, however; he is part of a culture half-way between East and West in which the boundaries of science are more loosely defined. He works in areas which few Western researchers have the opportunity to investigate.

Tjarkovsky, like most self-motivated people, generally carries out his research alone and on a small scale. Even though his ideas are slowly gaining acceptance, he has few opportunities to test them out within an institutional framework. As this book makes clear, childbirth in the Soviet Union takes place under comparatively primitive conditions. Despite this, Tjarkovsky's deliveries are extremely successful. The unique photographs, taken from amateur films of Igor's work, demonstrate with sensitive intensity that human beings can enter the world in a new way and live joyfully and confidently in our element of origin – water.

This book, which deals with visions and opportunities, is not a scientific study in the classical sense. The author chose to make *Water Babies* a reportage – personal, inquiring, investigative. The book offers no definite answers, no ready-made methods. Igor Tjarkovsky's work shows us that all routes towards development are not closed. His theory that we must learn to live in our element of origin – water – in order to develop our full potential opens up new prospects for human life on earth.

I   'These newborns are

really swimming'

I've seen the films and the colour photographs. I've read newspaper articles in many languages about the newborn babies who can swim. I've spoken to people who are qualified to know and who assure me that it really is possible.

Nevertheless, it feels strange to be standing here, chest-high in lukewarm water in a swimming pool in Moscow. All around me, babies and children are splashing, swimming and diving. The oldest ones amuse themselves by climbing up on to the edge of the pool only to jump, with delighted shrieks, back into the water again. There they dive like small otters, staying underwater for long periods of time.

The younger children, under a year old, are not such skilful swimmers. They prefer to stay near an adult, though as much under the surface as above it. The very smallest are taken care of by an adult who calmly and rhythmically dips them under the surface of the water for several seconds at a time. They are also given specially constructed baby bottles to suck on underwater.

The liveliest youngster in the pool is Kostja, a three-year-old with well-developed muscles and precise, controlled

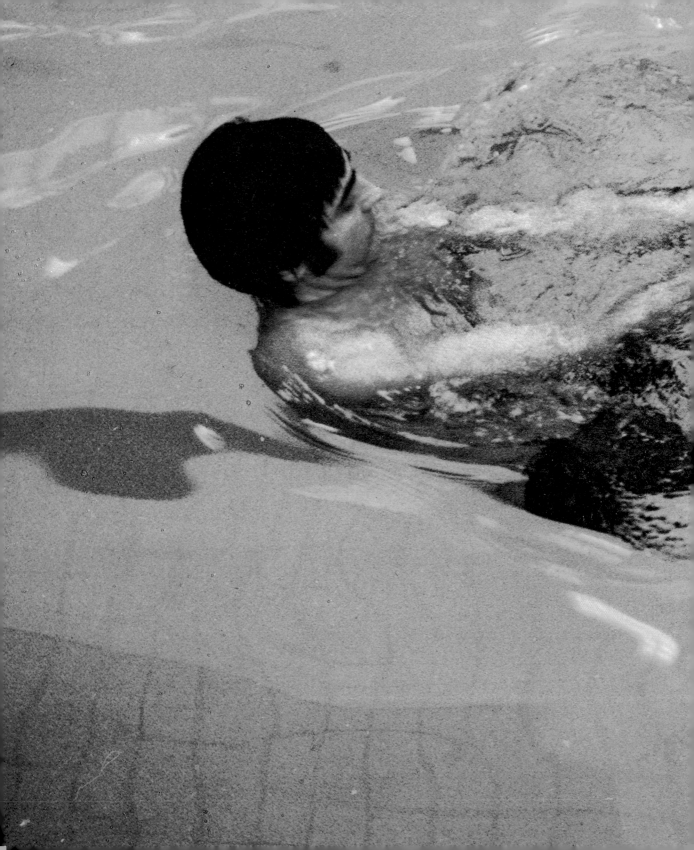

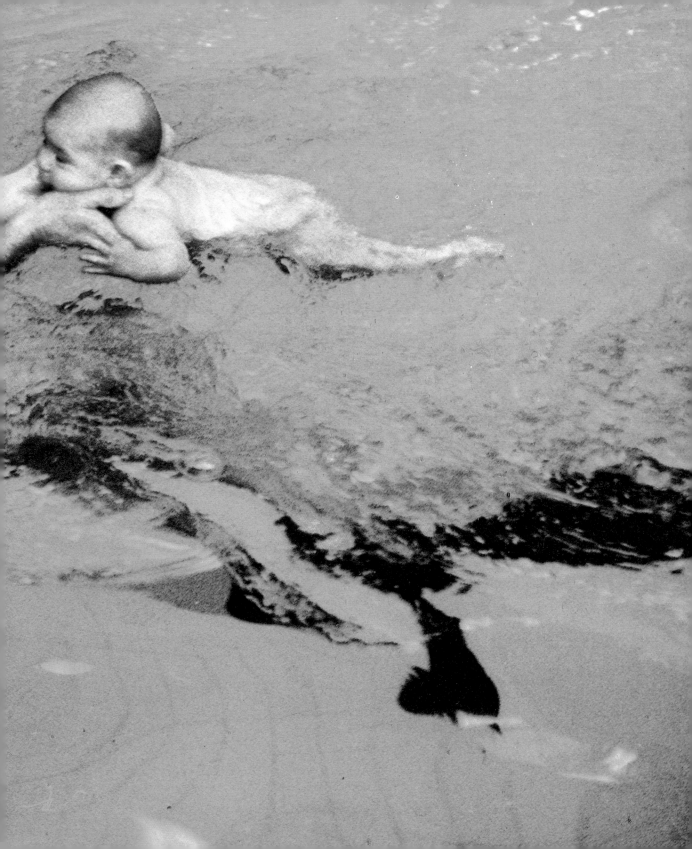

movements – truly athletic, if one can use the description of a young child. He is serious and self-possessed, but at the moment extremely jealous of Daddy's attention; Daddy is not to play with little brother Kolja, eight months old. Daddy has to swim with me.

'Daddy' is Igor Tjarkovsky, the Soviet researcher, pioneer of baby-swimming, who created a sensation with his photographs of swimming and diving newborns, and who aroused the interest of scientists with his theories about the significance of life in water for child development.

Here in the pool he is in his true element. He handles the children firmly but with great tenderness. He teaches the parents how to dip their children, how to play with them and coax them to stay underwater without fear.

The youngest child in the pool is Masja, two months old. When we met her outside with her parents, before training, she was swaddled in blankets like the Christ Child in a fresco – an orange parcel bound with red ribbons, the edge of a sheet and the tip of her nose poking out at one end.

Now she is totally unrestricted. Igor dips her in the water several times, then suddenly hands her over to me saying 'You saw how to do it'.

Taken by surprise, I stand holding her against my chest. Her mother, standing by the side of the pool, smiles at me encouragingly. Hesitantly, I say 'doo-doo-doo' to Masja, as Igor did. I hold her under the armpits, draw her down under the water, then in towards my body and up out of the water. Then I say 'doo-doo-doo' again, dip, draw in and up. Over and over again. She whimpers a little, but I understand that it is mainly because I am unfamiliar, not because she is being dipped in the water. She gazes at me all the while with large eyes through the clear water. It feels very strange.

The slightly older children love to jump in from the side of the pool. They return again and again to the water, where they feel completely at home.

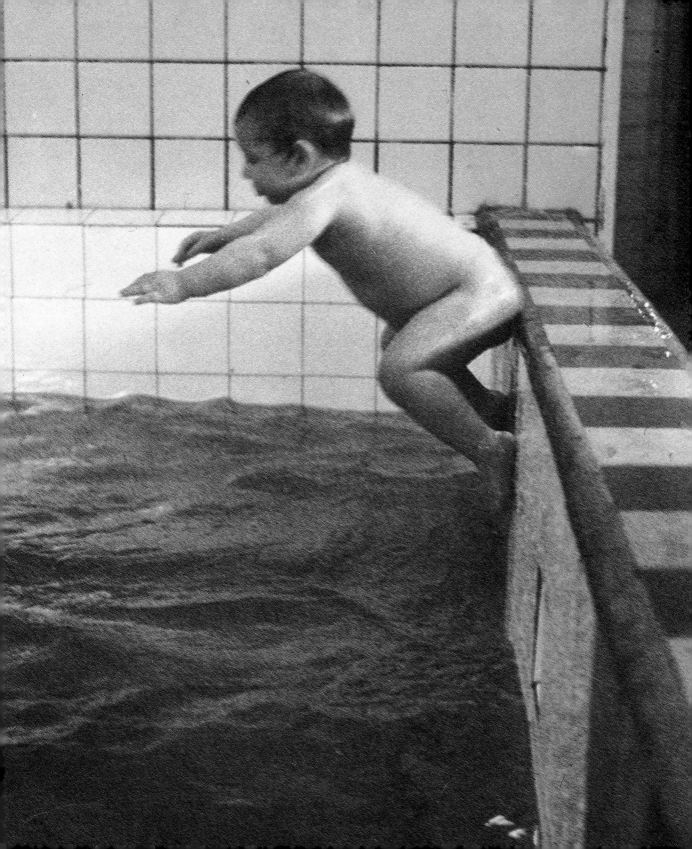

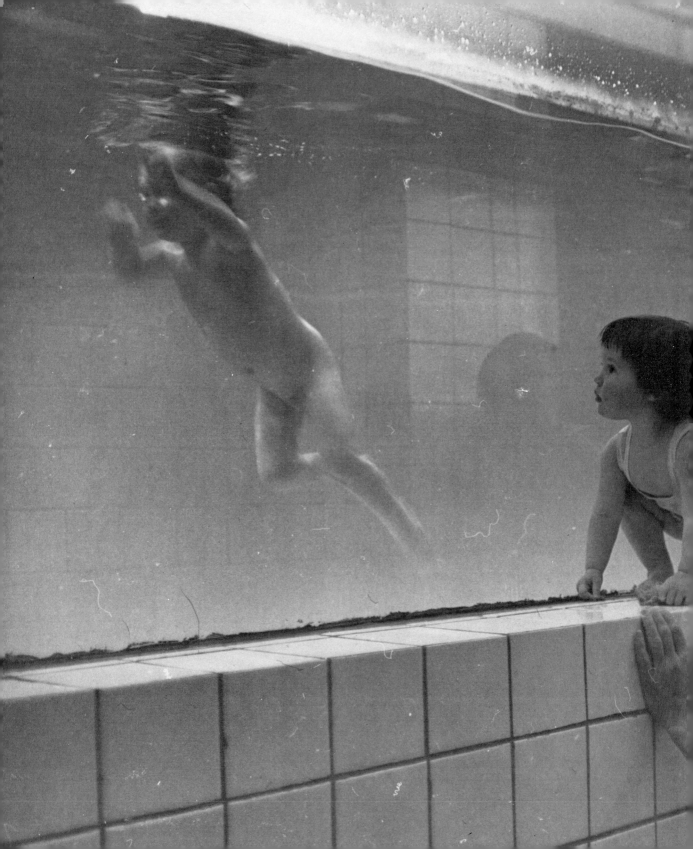

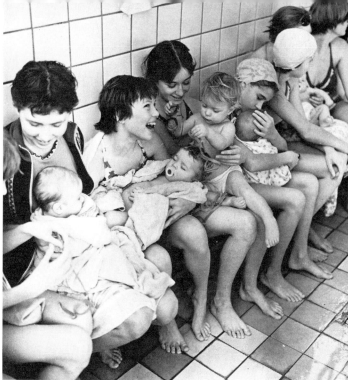

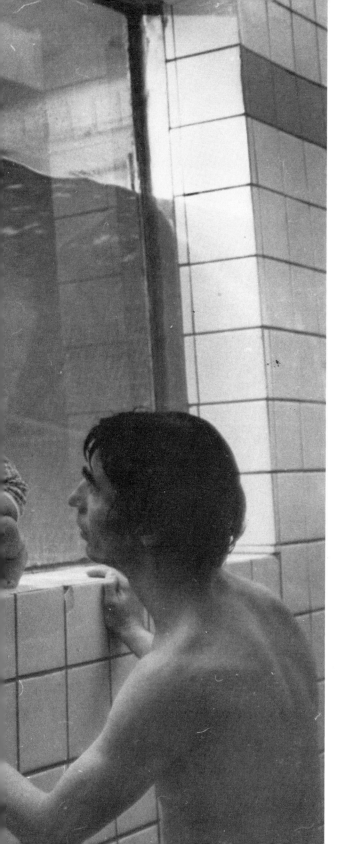

After a few hours in the pool, the children are tired and relaxed and often fall asleep in an adult's lap.

Other children can look through the observation window and see how their friends make their way through the water.

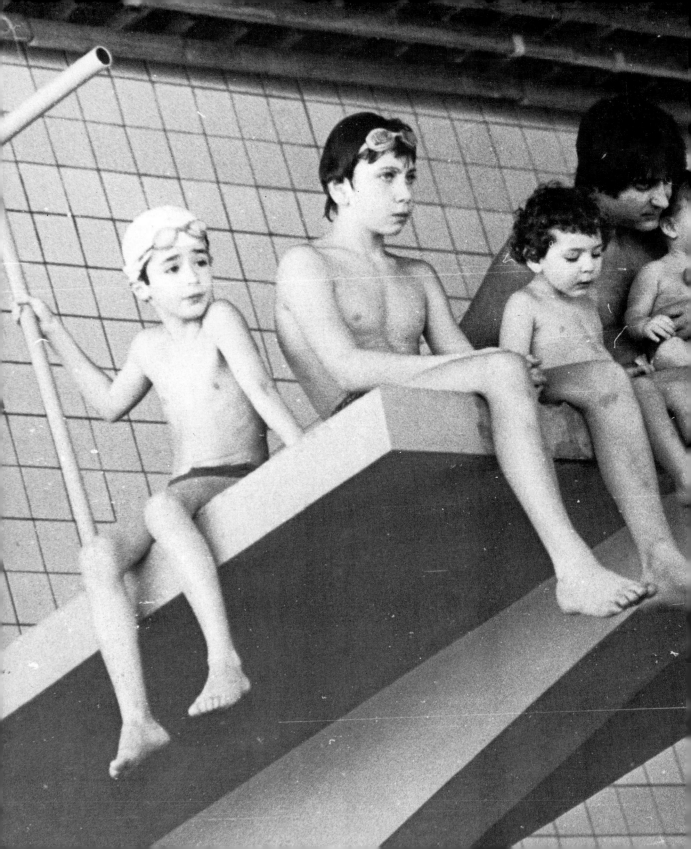

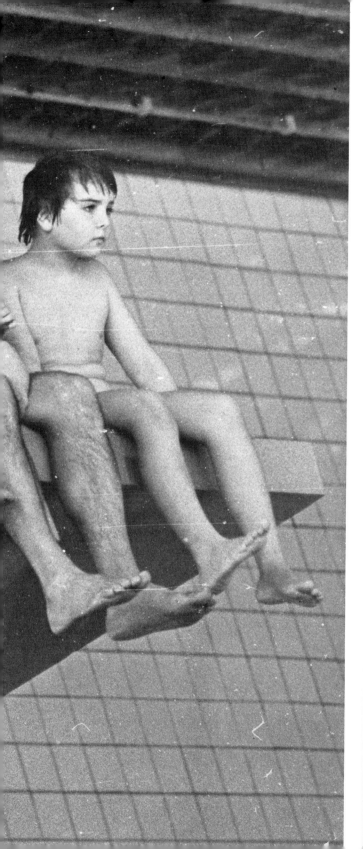

*Children of all ages gather
eagerly around Igor when he
comes to the pool. The
children who can swim also
like to dive, both from the
three-metre and the five-
metre-boards.*

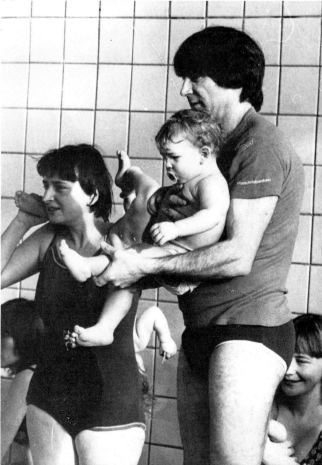

The air is warm and moist, the glass walls completely fogged up. Through them one catches a glimpse of frozen trees and the steam from the outdoor swimming pool. It is a cold day by the Moscow river. Here in the pool, parents and children romp noisily.

In Sweden and other Western countries, baby-swim has become a popular family pastime, an enjoyable and relaxing physical activity which brings together parents and children, helps children adjust to water, and strengthens their bodies and resistance.

For Igor Tjarkovsky, however, what is happening here in the pool is part of something much larger.

'What you are seeing here is a new kind of people, the children of the Ocean,' says Igor seriously. 'Human development has been at a standstill for many thousands of years; has reached an impasse. A life in water opens up new possibilities for development.'

Many years of assiduous scientific work and research lie behind the children's happy, carefree splashing in the pool: studies and theory-building; experiments with animals and practical application of the results to children; patient, tireless work with parents and children. He has a single-minded perseverance, a firm belief in his own ideas and an enthusiasm which has persuaded parents to come to him with their children.

We meet in the changing-room after training. Parents dry off their children, search for misplaced socks and attempt to open jammed lockers.

Little Masja lies on her stomach on a bench, covered with a thin terry towel. Her mother sees to it that she doesn't roll off, while taking the opportunity to massage her back gently. Masja has coughed up a little water and lies sniffling. I gaze at her thoughtfully, wondering if this is what a person of the future looks like.

This is what Igor believes. Simply, that water training allows the child to develop in ways which were never possible for the rest of us.

For several reasons, newborns can in water make better and more full use of the early, extremely receptive period of their lives.

If the child is also born underwater, it is given an extra-good start in life. Igor claims that sudden exposure at birth to the force of gravity after months of weightlessness in the womb, and a sudden, huge dose of oxygen taken in with the very first breath, are two elements which affect the most sensitive brain functions.

A gentle transition, both to the world of gravity and to a different way of breathing, opens up completely new possibilities for the human race.

'We are not confronting the child with anything new. We are simply prolonging the uterine conditions so beneficial to development. Living in water is totally natural for a

Parents and children romp and play in the pool. This allows close physical contact and provides important training, says Igor Tjarkovsky.

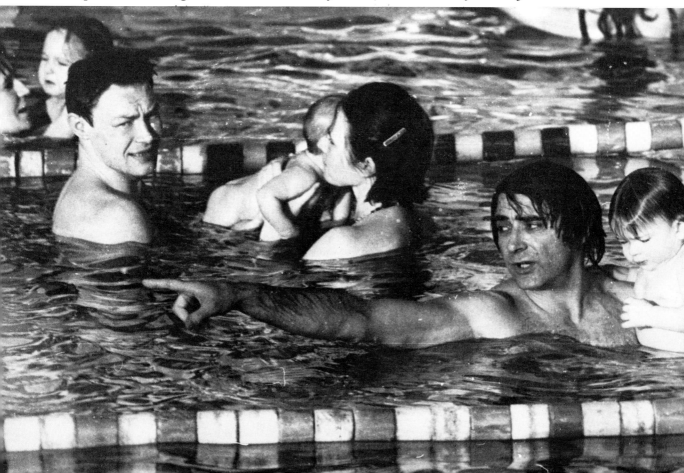

newborn. He's never done anything else . . . '

'What's your reaction to what you've seen today?' asks Igor. I answer incoherently that it has been interesting and bewildering.

'I want you to know that this was not a "good" day in the pool – it never is when outsiders are present. The children sense the disturbance. You are not only a stranger to them, a new face, but they can also sense the doubt and fear you most probably feel. "What if they drown!"

All of these things must be taken into consideration when working with waterbabies. We have a great deal to talk about.'

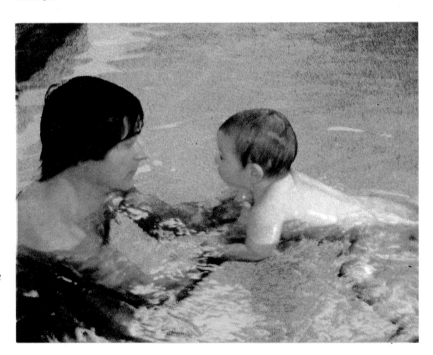

Igor, swimming with his son Kostya, provides a model for other parents.

2

Some news concerning childbirth

'Babies born underwater! Who eat, swim and dive under-water! It is to find out more about something so incredible that I have come to Moscow.'

I sit in my hotel room, gazing out over the enormous, haze-covered city. What are they all talking about? Is it fantastically interesting or simply fantastic? Shall I accept it or reject it?

I decide not to take a stand for the time being. Simply take in what I see, make a note of what I hear. Something will have to give eventually.

Deliver a child underwater? How absurd! one might think. But wouldn't an eighteenth-century woman have said the same thing about the way a twentieth-century woman gives birth? Lying on her back in front of a male doctor who listens with his ear pressed to her stomach to what is going on inside her instead, as the custom then was, of sitting on a chair or kneeling, surrounded by other women and perhaps a wise old healer-woman?

New movements have already been made, however. Absurd they may be – but during the last few decades there have been a number of innovations in the area of childbirth.

One of the first to challenge the attitude that childbirth was exclusively the hospital's concern ('Don't scream now, Mrs. Smith, it will get much worse later on') was the English doctor Grantly Dick-Read, who during the 'thirties launched a technique called 'Birth without fear'.

In the 'sixties, the method known as psychoprophylaxis (natural childbirth) was introduced. This method not only effectively reduces pain, it also reintroduces a different expectation: that the mother should actively participate in the delivery of her child.

Psychoprophylaxis was invented by a Soviet physician named Nikolajev. It is not in use in the Soviet Union today (where, incidentally, the techniques of childbirth could be greatly improved, according to many reports). From the Soviet Union the method soon reached France, where it was popularized by a doctor named Lamaze, and quickly spread to many other parts of the world.

The Lamaze method influenced Frederick Leboyer, another Frenchman who had a great impact upon our view of childbirth. 'Birth without violence' was his motto. He maintained that the newborn child must be received gently into the world, and the transition from the womb made as gentle as possible with subdued lighting, calm voices, soft hands and a warm bath after cutting the cord.

Leboyer has a follower in France called Michel Odent. He advocates (and carries out in practice) that the woman herself be allowed to sense and choose the way in which she would like to deliver, whether it is on all fours, squatting, on a chair, in a bed or in a water-filled tank.

28

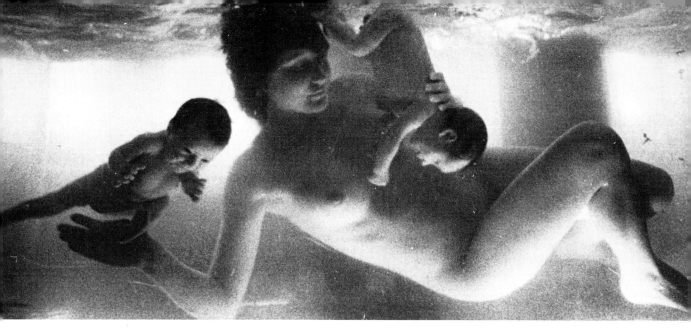

There are interesting similarities between Igor Tjarkovsky and Michel Odent, even if their work has different theoretical bases.

Michel Odent began using the tank of water for its relaxing and anaesthetic effect upon the mother, but soon discovered that it was possible to give the baby a gentle start in life by delivering it in water.

Michel Odent has, like Igor, experienced water's almost miraculous powers. He too speaks of the way in which a woman, during labour, enters into an altered, meditative state if treated gently, allowed to listen to her own inner signals and shape her own delivery.

The women who give birth under Igor's guidance often describe similar experiences.

Psychoprophylaxis, on the other hand, is if anything anti-meditative. Emphasis is placed on *not* losing contact with the surroundings, not letting go, and keeping the consciousness clear the entire time. Psychoprophylaxis's breathing technique also increases the oxygen level of the blood, which is not one of Igor's goals.

But, after the delivery, newborns who can swim? This

'Water-mother'. Like a water-goddess of ancient mythology, the woman rests with her infants in the element where all of life originates.

29

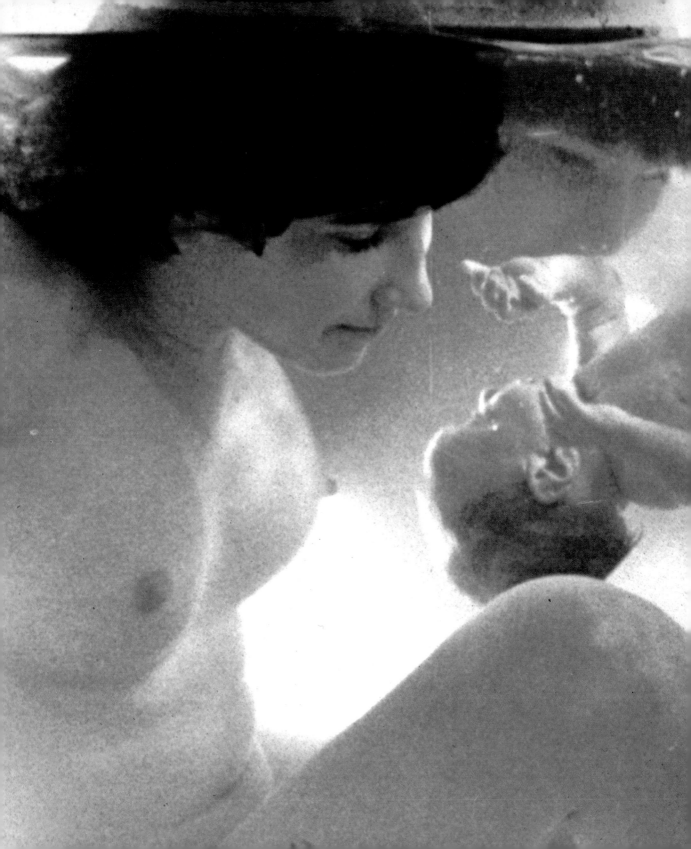

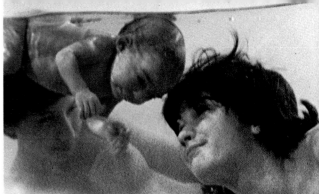

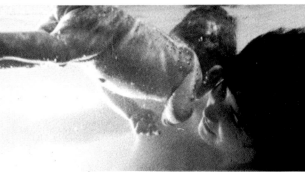

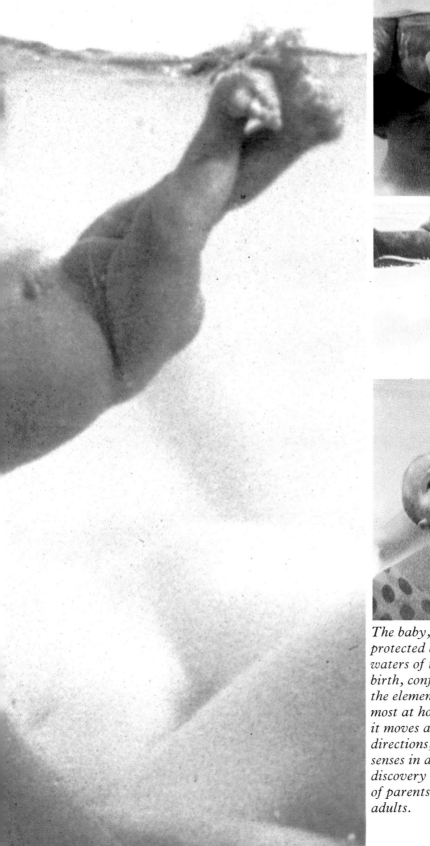

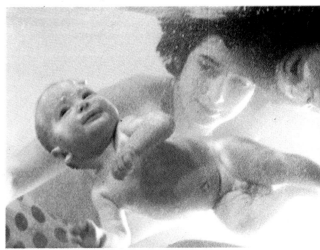

The baby, just as secure and protected as it was in the waters of the womb, can, after birth, confidently investigate the element in which it feels most at home. With open eyes, it moves around in all directions, uses its limbs and senses in a playful voyage of discovery under the supervision of parents and other trained adults.

sensational idea made headlines in newspapers and magazines.

West Germany is one of the countries in which there has been the most research and progress. At the Institute for Athletic Studies in Cologne, research has been underway since the 'sixties, and in Sweden researchers are investigating the possible benefits of 'baby-swim'.

In the Soviet Union, baby-swimming is encouraged and carried out widely under the motto 'swim first – walk second'.

Igor Tjarkovsky is critical of this development, however. He believes that it is superficial, and that a sense of the whole has been lost through concentration on a detail.

3

'Life has its origins in water'

I meet Igor again the next day. I know that he has carried out his research at the institution called, in the heavy Soviet vocabulary, 'The All-Union Scientific Research Institute for Physical Culture'.

We do not meet there, however, but in a cosy private apartment over glasses of hot tea with fragrant, golden cherry preserves. It is pleasant here and less strained than in a cold, impersonal office. I have realized, however, that Igor has a number of problems in his association with the Institute – even if he does not give the slightest hint of this.

'Water is the cradle of life here on earth. Life originated in the ocean more than three billion years ago. Somewhere in the warm seas, the first primitive creatures were formed, increased in number, developed. At long last, creatures began crawling on land. The sea had become overpopulated and some animals found fit to leave it in search of new living space, in flight from enemies.

There, for the first time, they were exposed to the force of gravity. The sea offers its inhabitants conditions approaching weightlessness. Emergence from the sea was thus a painful and difficult process. That short step from the water up on to solid land meant a many-million-year-long duel between the living creatures and the force of gravity.

Life on earth has its origins in water even today. Mammals and human beings spend their first months of life in water, floating in warm weightlessness. They are protected from the harshness of the outside world, in close contact with the mother, with her thoughts and feelings.

We have always known that the foetus develops in water in the womb. We have been able to observe this, both during our own deliveries and those of animals.

It is also obvious that water will support an object dropped into it. Archimedes two thousand years ago formulated exactly how the process works. But even the cavemen knew through experience what Archimedes's principle implied. All they had to do was fall into the water.

Newton formulated the law of gravity a mere three hundred years ago. But even the very earliest animals knew that gravity was nothing to play around with. They were aware of it whenever they had to leap over a gorge.

Gravity doesn't only affect falling bodies, however. Its influence reaches to all parts of life. Even the development and functioning of every tiny cell is subject to its force.

There is one element on our earth, however, in which gravity does not make its presence felt to the same degree: water. Even if weightlessness in water is not total, water still provides a refuge from gravity's death-blow.

The water in which the foetus develops protects it from injury. Take an egg yolk, for example. Break it on to a plate and it flattens out, collapses. Break it into a glass of water instead, and it retains its form. The same principle applies to a newborn baby's brain. The tissues around it are not much stronger than the membrane around an egg yolk.

Another property of water also facilitates foetal development. When the organism is not exposed to the force of gravity, its need for oxygen decreases by 60–75%. Much less of the available oxygen is thus needed for maintenance of bodily functions, and a larger portion can be used for growth, development and renewal of organs, bones and muscles.'

'I have personally experienced the healing properties of water', Igor continues. 'It happened by chance several years ago. I was swimming alone in the pool, on my back, and I must have misjudged the distance to the edge of the pool. I drove my head into it with full force. The result was a full-blown concussion. I was unconscious for several hours – I could verify this when I came to. I had lain floating in the water the entire time. Nobody was aware of my accident.

I could scarcely breathe. Every breath I drew pounded painfully in my head. Gradually the pain began to subside and I could breathe more deeply. At last I was able to get out of the water and actually felt all right.

I've had concussions before, so I'm aware of the long and difficult convalescence period which can follow. This time, however, because I lay in the water, I was practically speaking restored to normal within a few hours.

Why, then, don't we utilize water's resources to a greater extent? Why have animals – and people – forgotten how to swim?' I asked.

'All creatures *can* swim', says Igor. 'All creatures can continue the life in water they were living before birth, as my numerous experiments with animals have shown.

My experiments have also shown, however, that all land animals have a deep-rooted fear of water. Even desert animals that have only seen water in the form of dew-drops display a terror of water which cannot possibly originate in

35

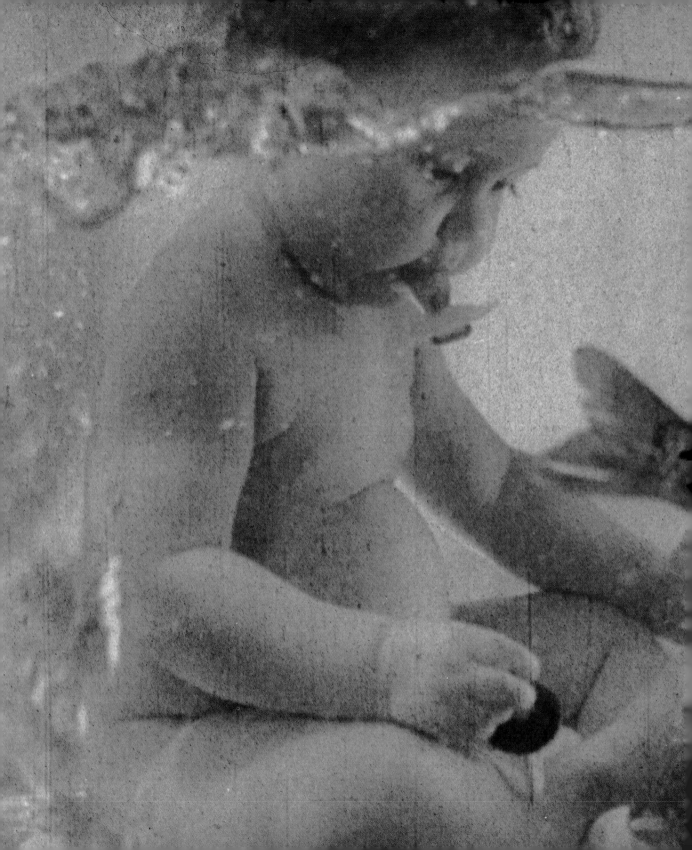

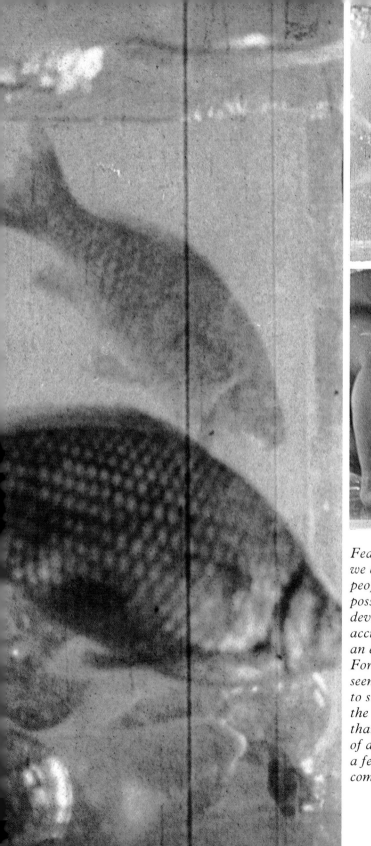

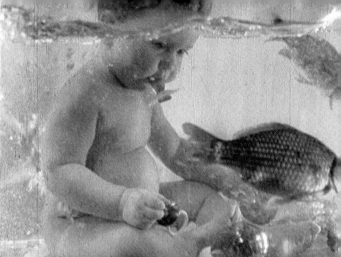

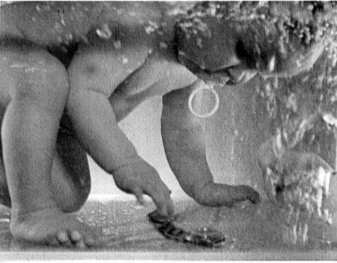

*Fear of water, which
we believe that all
people naturally
possess, need never
develop if babies grow
accustomed to water at
an early age.
For this little girl, it
seems no more unusual
to sit and play under
the water's surface
than above it. Instead
of a cat or dog, she has
a few fish to keep her
company.*

their own experience.

I prefer to regard this universal fear of water as a genetic memory, an inheritance from the time when our animal forefathers left the sea to become land animals. In order to survive the new conditions, they were forced to develop a new form of energy maintenance, a new physiology suited to movement on land; to alter completely the structure of the body and develop an incredibly complex nervous system. One condition for achieving all this was never to return to the sea. It had been abandoned once and for all.

The weak could not survive these new conditions. The strong continued the fight for survival on land, guided by the instinct stamped into them by this evolutionary process. There could be no way back. The sea was full of enemies, predators ready to devour any creature who attempted to break the line of evolution and return. Gravity was a tough opponent, but the fear of the monsters in the sea was stronger.

But these sea-monsters died out millions of years ago! you protest. No, not completely. They still exist in the sub-conscious mind of every land animal, ready to swallow us up should we try to return.

This fear of the monsters in the sea has become the "common sense" which declares my research and theories to be nonsense. It is a very real dread, however, which can paralyse human beings in their encounters with water and which prevents us from making full use of the opportunities this element offers us. And remember, water covers two-thirds of the earth's surface.

Why do people drown? Not because they can't swim. A relaxed person will float without swimming a stroke. It is *fear* which paralyses us, fear against which even a powerful swimmer is helpless.

This fear can be unlearned, however, It takes several months for fear to "connect" in the baby's brain, before it is reinforced, confirmed by the parents' own dread. Consciously and unconsciously, we transmit our fear to the new generation. I believe that we also transmit this fear telepathically.

I have devoted the greater part of my life to demonstrating, in theory and in practice, that people can acquire a new attitude towards water, and that our inherited fear of water can be unlearned. This is what my work in the swimming pool is all about.

My reason for wanting to work in this area is my firm conviction that it provides the key to the continued mental and physical development of the human race.'

'Igor, how long have you been involved with these issues?' I asked.

'Actively since the beginning of the 'sixties, in my mind even earlier. At times I've made rapid progress, at times I've merely spun my wheels. This is probably typical of all scientific work.

One problem I've run up against in my work is that releasing information during the experimental stages can arouse extremely negative reactions and even result in medical authorities feeling obliged to intervene and stop the experiments.

On the other hand, if one carries out experiments without allowing outside observation, and only displays finished results (newborns who can swim), experts will demand proof before they can believe what they see with their own eyes.

It's a vicious circle. One can't work openly because then the whole enterprise will be classed as criminal, and one can't convince others of the authenticity of the results if they haven't followed the development step by step.'

'It sounds as if you are speaking from personal experience.'

'Yes. I was forced to break off a series of experiments with sickly and premature babies which I was carrying out at a children's home. Those in charge supported my attempts to improve the children's strength and physical abilities through organized water training, and I had begun to achieve fine results. But information about my activities began to leak out and many people considered what I was doing to be on a par with torture. The administration was forced to yield to the pressure.

As early as 1962, our Institute for Physical Culture supported studies of children's swimming ability. Professional female swimmers participated with their babies and young children. This was the first time we experimented with underwater nursing, among other things. We kept our results secret, however. Neither the general public nor the scientific establishment was ready for them. It was not possible for the Institute to publish our findings. This could have led to negative reactions and, presumably, the imposition of bans by medical authorities.

Journalists were not given information about our experiments, either. But a year later, in 1963, I wrote a cautious internal report for the Institute.

During the following years, a number of films were shown for researchers and midwives. One of the films, which showed a baby diving for a bottle, aroused violently negative reactions among doctors and midwives.

Despite the adverse publicity, I did receive a great deal of moral support from prominent scientists such as the biologist Michail Ivanitski and Dr. Nikolaj Bernstein, a fellow in the Soviet Academy of Medicine (he had been curious about the "meaningless" movements which newborns make – I was able to show him that they were swimming strokes). Bernstein's successor as director of the Sports and Bio-mechanics Laboratory of the Institute for Physical Culture, Ivan Ratov, allowed me to use the laboratory facilities and I carried out many of my experiments there.

My attempts to collaborate with various medical research institutions, on the other hand, led nowhere, despite a growing conviction on the part of many obstetricians and paediatricians that treatment of premature babies in water could be beneficial.'

4   It's safe

to go in water

'I had a theory,' says Igor. 'Or rather, two theories. First, as to how the organism is affected by not being exposed to the force of gravity and second, as to how land animals, including man, can adapt to a life in water.

I've tested my theories on animals, and then gone on to work with humans. With children, we have only been able to do 10% of the work that was possible with animals.

I have worked with many kinds of animals: cockroaches, mice, chickens, rabbits, cats and many others, and I can assure you that a cockroach is a great deal wiser than a professor. The cockroach learns after only a few minutes that it is perfectly safe to go into the water, whereas the professor may never learn. His prejudices are so ingrained in him that he finds it impossible to believe what he sees with his own two eyes. But the cockroach can reconsider the matter.

Not until I had done thousands of experiments with animals did I begin to understand what kind of problem I was attempting to solve. Up to then I hadn't really realized how deep down in the unconscious mind of all land animals – including man – the fear of water lies. I could never have dreamed of the complex ties which exist between different sides of the problem, of the subtleness with which our ancestors control our way of viewing the world, or of the forces in the battle between old and new in our way of thinking.

My experiments with animals showed me just how deep-rooted and tenacious this fear of water is. Mice preferred to stay near a cat rather than escape through a tunnel which they had previously been accustomed to using but which had now been filled with water.

My experiments also showed, however, that this fear can be unlearned – something of which I had actually been aware since childhood. I once found a little kitten that someone had left in a rubbish bin to die. I must have washed it at least a hundred times in a bucket to get rid of the loathsome smell. I noticed that the kitten quite soon had no problem coping with water. It was completely unafraid and seemed to enjoy all the washing.

Later, however, when I began experimenting with animals, I discovered that the normal reaction of adult cats is totally different. They would fight desperately against any attempts made to place them in water. If I was too persistent, they experienced serious stress and could even die.

The same was true for other land animals: hens, pigs or monkeys.

Eventually, however, it proved possible, with special training, to free the animals from their fear of water, mainly with the help of food.

We began very simply. For example, we placed grains of corn in a dish, filled it with water and placed it in front of a hen. In order to get at the corn, the hen was forced to stick her beak into the water – but nothing else. This was something which the hen could handle.

Step by step we made the tasks more difficult – part of her head had to be dipped into the water, and so on.

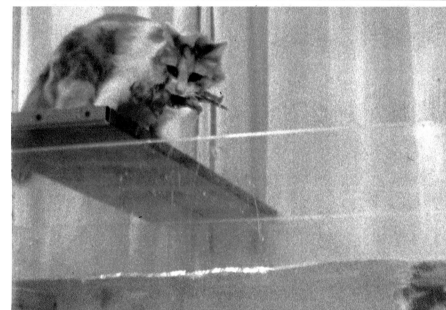

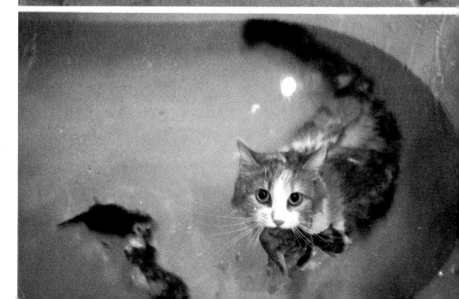

Cats are generally afraid of water. With adequate training and positive reinforcement they can become 'water animals', able to deliver their young in water without fear.

After completing this course the various animals could stay in the water for hours at a time, picking up food from the bottom. It also became apparent that the positive stimulation which food provided brought about a direct improvement in various performances. One example: kittens that dived underwater to nurse could hold their breath five times longer than when they were forced to dive.

The interesting thing, however, was that under certain circumstances animals not only entered the water without fear but also brought their offspring with them, and in certain cases even gave birth in the water.

A monkey that had learned to stay in the water for hours at a time, picking up food from the bottom, continued to do so when she'd had a baby. The youngster would sit clinging tightly to her back, and had soon learned to nurse underwater. By the time it was fully grown it had adapted perfectly to a life in water.

At times we noticed that our experiments with young animals were not so successful if the mother was present. We came to the conclusion that she transmitted her own fear of water to her offspring and that a water animal could, on the other hand, transmit a sense of security. For example, chicks were calm in the water with a duck nearby.

This is a very important point when it comes to working with waterbabies. The training and preparation of the expectant mother is directed towards precisely this problem. I shall discuss this point in depth later on.

An account of all the experiments we have carried out would fill several books. But the gist of our findings is as follows.

1. All animals can adapt to a life in water.
2. All animals can give birth in water.
3. All animals can raise their young in water.

The natural conclusion one draws from all this is that human beings ought to be capable of the same things.

But why? you ask. What are the advantages of living in water?

Many, I assure you! Life did not originate in water merely by chance, nor is it coincidence that the foetus floats in water during the most important stages of its development. I shall discuss this at greater length, but while we're on the subject of experimentation with animals, we may as well begin with those experiments demonstrating the way in which weightlessness in water influences oxygen requirements.

I mounted a glass globe with the opening downwards in a tank of water. In this way, animals could swim into the globe without surfacing.

With the help of this globe, I was able to observe the way in which the animals' oxygen consumption decreased in water. Inside the globe I placed a raft with various types of small animals as passengers. For other animals of the same species I had constructed special small life-belts which enabled them to float with their heads above the surface of the water. By and by the oxygen in the globe began to run out. The animals on the raft showed clear signs of discomfort and eventually lost consciousness. The animals afloat in the water, however, endured the lack of oxygen without visible problem.

I conducted a similar experiment with two pregnant rabbits, whose labour had begun. I placed one on "dry land" in a glass globe with a low oxygen level. Her labour ceased almost immediately and she fell into a coma. The bottom half of the other globe was filled with water, and here I placed the second rabbit. Her delivery proceeded normally in the water.

This change in oxygen requirements has been demonstrated by several other researchers.

Water-dwelling mammals switch over to a different type of metabolism underwater. It requires less oxygen than the normal form, known as glycolysis, in which carbohydrates are broken down in the musculature.

In 1959, a report was published on seals' ability to stay underwater for more than twenty minutes at a time. As soon as the seal ducks its head under water its pulse rate decreases by approximately 90% to between 10 and 12 beats per minute.

A large portion of the blood circulation is cut off so that the blood levels around the heart and brain are remarkably low. Through use of radioactive isotopes, which do not reach the muscles and only penetrate the inner organs to a very slight degree, it can be demonstrated that the waste products formed in glycolysis remain in the muscles.

As soon as the seal pokes its head up out of the water, however, its blood circulation returns to normal. The waste products are washed out of the muscles, oxidized with oxygen from the air and leave the body via the lungs.

Human begins also have this potential from birth, and it can be maintained through training.

All handbooks on the art of delivery say that a newborn baby can survive without breathing for ten to fifteen minutes as opposed to an adult who can only survive for two to three minutes. (Some newborns have actually managed an hour at birth without oxygen supply, and it also appears that premature babies are less vulnerable than others to a lack of oxygen.)

This "water mammal function" can thus be maintained in humans with the help of water training. (It can also disappear in water animals who are kept out of the water.)

Water training also enables us to retain the reflex which closes off the windpipe underwater, and the ability to swim which all newborns possess. (Their movements resemble an adult's breaststroke, but are more perfect and automatic. The adult has learned how to swim; the baby has never forgotten.)

Our experiments with animals have also shown the long-

48

term effects of an upbringing in water upon land animals. Compared with "normal" animals of the same species, animals raised in water proved to be more well-developed in several ways.

Pigs raised in water were larger and stronger. Rabbits raised by beavers were not only more powerfully built, but their life expectancy doubled. The same was true for other animals.

We also observed that the animals raised in water produced better and quicker results on intelligence tests.

Naturally, one should not jump to conclusions concerning human beings. But fascinating perspectives certainly open for the waterbabies.

There is nothing strange about it. All the energy which on land is used to fight the force of gravity is freed in water. What is it used for instead?

1. To develop the body, and above all the brain.

2. To investigate the environment and acquire different kinds of knowledge.

3. To create new brain functions which will enable people to solve problems and handle tasks which are impossible for those of us born and raised in the normal, handicapped way.

It's really only a question of allowing the wonder of human development to unfold without interruption. The development of the brain's structure doesn't begin at birth. It has started much earlier, in the womb. We now know that this same development can continue after birth, uninterrupted.

"What happens afterwards, though? Aren't we just postponing the matter? The child has to go on land sooner or later," say the critics, and believe they've produced an unassailable argument. But they have not.

Research has shown that newborns are not the passive bundles they were previously thought to be. Even during their first few hours they are capable of receiving great amounts of information, of discovering the world and the people around them. The earlier water training can be started the better, since newborns are so tremendously open and receptive.

With my method, maximum use can be made of this early, receptive and active period.

First of all, delivery in water protects the baby's brain from the strain and possible damage inflicted upon it by a sudden transition to the world of gravity.

Second, the baby has much more energy to spend on developing its body and brain, energy which would otherwise be used to fight the force of gravity.

Third, the baby's weightlessness in water allows it to move about freely in three dimensions and discover the world around it. Instead of lying flat on its back in a basket, perhaps lifting its head to stare at a plastic toy, the child in water can turn, dive, lie on its stomach and back and use its limbs.

And all this during the first weeks and months when the child's receptivity and potential for development are so great. It is an opportunity which will never return. Can one really say, then, as my critics do, that it is simply a matter of postponement?

By the age of three months, "my" children are at the ability level of a normal one-year-old. They are also extremely strong and physically well-developed, and therefore well-equipped to handle life on land.

We know that the foetus develops in water in the womb because water provides the most beneficial environment possible for development. What could be more reasonable than prolonging these beneficial conditions for a time?

I've treated handicapped children in water, children with atrophied muscles who could not sit or stand. In the water they could move around and function just like healthy, normal children of the same age.

I consider such a child a challenge. If water can give this child life and strength, imagine what it can do for a child born with full resources.'

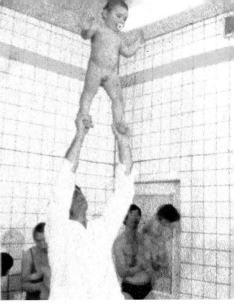

Parents who have swum with their babies meet in the bathhouse after training. They proudly show off their own tadpoles and admire other children's abilities.

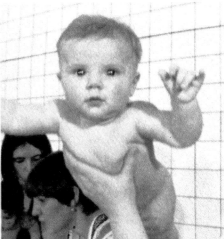

A water-trained child can also see clearly under water. Here, Igor holds up a book and the boy gazes eagerly at the pictures.

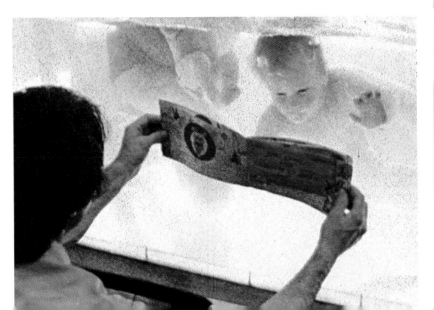

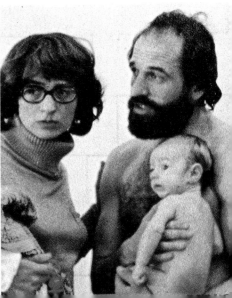

5   'I can't

help asking'

'Igor Tjarkovsky, who are you? How did you come to devote your life to this work?'

'I was born in the Urals forty-five years ago, but spent part of my youth in Altaj, near the Siberian–Mongolian border. There I first came into contact with traditional "healers", people who can use their energy to heal and influence others. There I also found the abandoned kitten which I've told you about.

Later, as an adult, I took a technical degree and worked as a boat-builder. I later changed careers and became an athletics coach. I have since built upon the latter qualification with studies in various fields, biology, psychology, and so on. I am also a qualified male midwife.

People often wonder who I really am, and what my specialty is. Since it is difficult to give an exact answer, many grow suspicious and doubt my scientific status.

I am not simply a biologist, doctor or athletics coach. I cannot say that I work in any specific field.

I've devoted the last twenty years of my life to solving the problem of how we can help newborns adjust to water's environment. This is a problem which cannot be restricted to any particular field, but which spans many areas of knowledge. It requires a comprehensive, overall view which not only encompasses the traditional sciences but also fringe subjects such as parapsychology.

The most exact description of the work I'm involved in would be "an investigation into the opportunities for developing human potential".

Once, during my studies, I came across a book in which the author objectively and in great detail described how excellent conditions in the womb are for the foetus, and how painful it is for a newborn to be subjected to the force of gravity which crushes fragile heads and kills weak and premature babies. On that occasion I simply scribbled angrily in the margin "deliver underwater, then!"

This was a natural reaction for me and I wondered why the author did not also react in this way.

Through the years, all the "whys" grew more and more numerous until I finally realized that in order to get any further in my work I'd have to find an answer to all these questions.

Why can't we deliver babies in water in order to spare them the painful transition from a state of near-weightlessness to the full effect of gravity's force?

Why do we place the victim of a traffic accident on a stretcher in a jolting ambulance in which the injuries are only aggravated, instead of in a water-filled tank which helps reduce both physical strain and energy requirements?

And above all, why do people drown? Every year, all over the world, approximately two hundred and fifty to three hundred thousand people drown. That's an average of one person every other minute.

Because they can't swim, you say. But all animals *can* swim, I have proved this scientifically. People drown

'To find a reasonable answer to all of my questions, I must adopt a holistic view of existence which spans many branches of science,' says Igor Tjarkovsky.

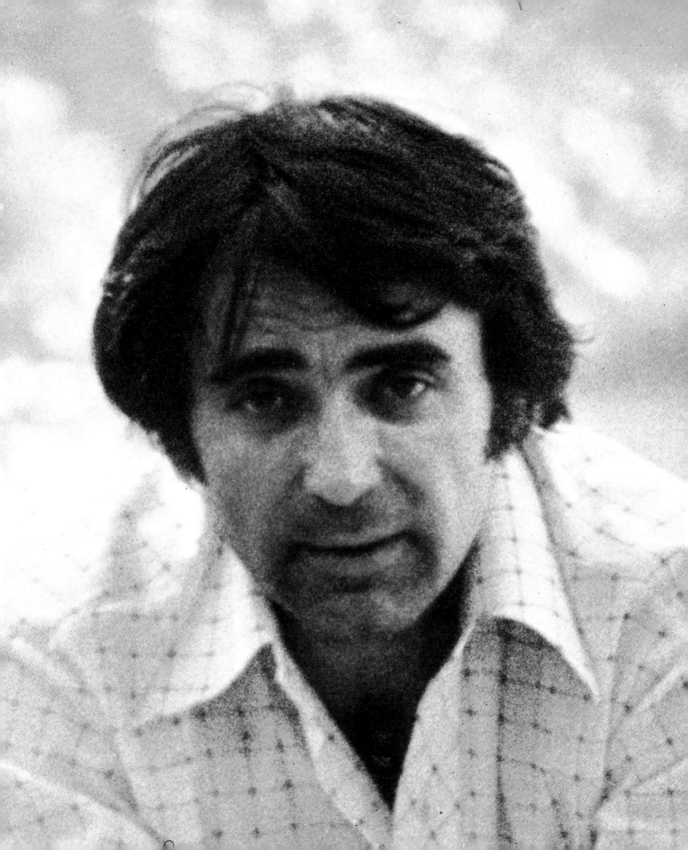

because they are afraid. This fear lies deep within the subconscious and, when it comes to the surface, it paralyzes both reason and will.

In 1962, while working as an athletics coach, I was confronted with a problem which challenged all my speculations.

My daughter Veta was born two months prematurely. She weighed only a little over two and a half pounds and was extremely weak and underdeveloped. The doctors at the hospital despaired of saving her life. I asked permission to take over responsibility for her care and they agreed.

I want to emphasize the fact that this was no experiment on my part. It was a desperate attempt to save the life of someone dear to me.

I placed Veta in a tub filled with ninety-three to ninety-five degree water. At first I kept the water level quite low – just high enough for her to lie on the bottom – but when I saw how well she was developing I grew bolder and added more water.

In the water, she could move her weak body more easily. She developed surprisingly rapidly and had soon caught up with her peers.

She ate nearly twice as much as other babies. At first, the doctors were afraid that she was being overfed, but had to concede that she was also much more active than other children.

I soon had to provide her with a larger tank in which she could swim and dive. The walls of the tank were transparent and I showed films and slides for her. I gave her live fish and frogs to play with. When she felt hungry, she would dive down and pick up a bottle that lay on the bottom of the tank.

She spent the greater part of her first two years in water. I only took her out of the tank when I was expecting visitors who might be shocked.

When she was seven months old I took her with me to the big outdoor swimming pool where I worked as a lifeguard. My chair was placed on a floating dock in the middle of the pool (the pool is divided into sections). After she had spent an hour in one section I would move her to a different one on the other side. In this way I could maintain a constant contact with her. Nobody else could understand, however, that she was perfectly content to lie floating in the water all day.

Sometimes I was able to take her with me to the big pool in the evenings and at night. I fastened a little lamp to her so that I could keep track of her whereabouts. She developed an amazing ability to orientate herself in the dark.

When she was two years old, I couldn't devote so much time to her and we were forced to cut down on the water training. By that time, however, she already looked like a four-year-old.

Veta was the first child to be raised in water in this way. Our appetites whetted by the success of this endeavour, my assistants and I carried out our first underwater delivery only a year later.

I too tried living in water. I spent a month in a shallow swimming pool where I ate, slept and worked on a scientific thesis. I only left the water to use the lavatory.

My, what energy I had! I really had resources to put into my work – I noticed that ideas and thoughts came to me much more easily than before. I also felt much stronger and more capable than those around me.

Before we continue, however, I'd like to point out that I have predecessors. Other researchers have made discoveries which have served as a starting-point for my own work.

Barcroft has demonstrated in various ways how the organism's oxygen requirements decrease in water. Legent-jenko and Sokolov discovered a good many years ago that

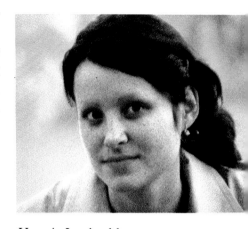

Veta is Igor's oldest daughter. She was born 20 years ago, two months prematurely. Her father saved her life by caring for her in a tub filled with lukewarm water. She developed surprisingly rapidly and had soon caught up with her peers. Through the years, Igor continued to water-train her. Veta, the first 'water baby', is today an independent, determined and harmonious young woman.

one can help weak newborns by bathing them for fifteen to twenty minutes after delivery. This is an effective method which has yet to be introduced in our maternity hospitals. It has probably seemed too simple to be taken seriously.

Kasmarskaja, the pathologist, has demonstrated that brain development proceeds more slowly outside the gravity-free environment of the womb. The brains of premature babies who died some time after birth have fewer nerve cells than the brain of a normally developed child of the same age, calculated from conception.

One of the most well-known researchers to have put forward the idea that the force of gravity imposes limits on the brain's development and thereby on human potential was Konstantin Tsiolkovsky. He maintained that human development will remain at a standstill until technology allows us to colonize space on a large scale. He had fantastic visions of how life in this gravity-free environment would radically alter the human condition.

But why wait for such a distant and uncertain future? Another element, much closer to us, can render us almost equally weightless, can signify just as much for our development.

I am convinced that people have been aware of this fact in bygone times. There is much evidence to show that people of the past had knowledge of water's healing powers. In many religions, water plays an important role in various rituals.

In ancient times, water was a symbol for both immortality and fertility. Ancient Greek myths tell of how the gods used water to ensure themselves of a protected eternal life.

Baptism is one of Christianity's most important sacraments – indeed, one of the most important initiation rites in all religions.

Ritual baths were part of the Eleusinian Mysteries and of the cults of Dionysus and Isis. Ceremonies with water were part of the cults of Egypt, Assyria, Babylonia and Palestine. Many rituals included immersion in water, which symbolized the end of a sinful life and the beginning of a new and virtuous one. In Ancient Egypt, children destined to be priests were even delivered in water – they were then considered to be a special category of people with a special relationship to the supernatural.

The rite of baptism is described in detail in *The Teachings of the Twelve Apostles*, an early Christian text from the first century A.D. The following advice is given: "Baptize, in the name of the Father, the Son and the Holy Ghost, in living, flowing water. If living water is not to be found take cold, if cold is not to be found take warm."

It is interesting to note that cold water is preferred over warm. I know from my own experience that cold water (especially ice-cold melted snow) has fantastic healing powers. It stimulates blood circulation and respiration much more effectively than does warm.

Immersing newborns in holes cut in the ice has been a custom in Russia for centuries. I myself have seen weak, premature babies revive after being placed in cold water until they were blue. They were then taken out, wrapped in warm clothing and placed near a fire. This was common practice among the healers in Central Asia where I spent my youth.

One can only guess at what lies behind such a fabulous revival. It is conceivable that the structure of melted snow is in some way more beneficial to a weakened organism than the structure of warm or boiled water. Perhaps the structure of melted snow harmonizes in some way with the organism's cell structure, and thus has a beneficial effect upon it. This is only a hypothesis, however.

I also believe that both the ancient Mystery priests and the faith healers of Central Asia possessed certain unique psychological – or rather parapsychological – abilities. At the very least they were aware of and mastered certain special techniques. In other words, they knew exactly what they were doing. . . .

There is every reason to believe that in ancient times, priests and holy men were aware of water's remarkable powers. They were probably also aware of how water could be used to attain what we call higher forms of consciousness, to make contact with higher powers.

Baptism's original purpose was probably to create a solid connection between the child and God – a contact which could endure for a lifetime. Our ancient Christian churches are often located in places believed to favour contact with the universe. The baptismal font's bowl-shaped form collects and concentrates energy, and the water, in which the child in former times was totally immersed, helps the child to partake of this cosmic energy.

The more religious texts I read, the more convinced I become of the power of these ancient water rites, and of the unique influence they had on the human psyche.

Today these rituals have in many ways been reduced to mere technical acts of purely symbolic significance. This is what has happened to most ceremonies practised today, especially in the West.

From many quarters, however, a clear tendency is emerging to revive ancient knowledge and restore to rituals their previous significance. This is not merely a reaction against nihilism or the "spiritual crisis" so much has been written about. These ancient customs probably contained more practical significance than has generally been thought. It is our modern civilization which has reduced them to symbols.

We are slowly becoming aware that without an understanding of this dimension, continued human development is practically speaking impossible. We must study ancient knowledge once again.

Traditional academic studies are not the answer, however. The knowledge we need can only be gained through direct experience of the value of these ancient truths, not through a rationalistic stocking-up of information.'

6   'Bio-energy is a factor

to be reckoned with'

Igor Tjarkovsky is careful to emphasize that he does not fit into any traditional scientific pigeonhole. He wants to offer a comprehensive, overall view. In the West, he would probably be ranked with those striving towards a holistic, alternative form of medicine and health care. As is the case in this movement, parapsychological thought is an integral part of Igor's work.

'When I began experimenting with underwater deliveries, I was assisted by people known in this country as "sensitives" – people with parapsychological abilities,' says Igor. 'Even if they weren't present during the actual delivery they were able, through use of their bio-energy, to keep the situation under control. Because they can perceive people's biofields, they were able to see or sense whether certain factors were unfavourable and advise me against continuing the delivery underwater.

I myself desired this help and sense of security in my work. Since sensitives are relatively rare beings, however, others must perhaps seek different solutions.'

What is Igor talking about? Sensitives? Biofields? Bio-energy? Before we continue, perhaps we should define his terms.

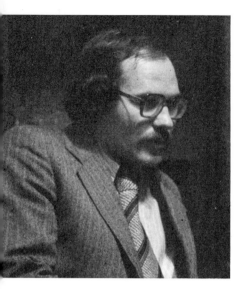

Bio-energy is one of many names for a form of energy in and around the human body. Many acknowledge its existence, but its physiological character has yet to be established.

This is the energy form which is affected by, among other things, Chinese acupuncture. Acupuncturists call it 'Chi'. Disturbances in the flow of this energy through the body can result in illness.

Certain religions and currents of ideas hold that bio-energy is of cosmic origin, that it pervades the entire universe and that life essentially amounts to a constant interchange of energy between all living creatures.

The bio-energy which surrounds the body is sometimes called the biofield. This field can be perceived – seen or sensed – by specially trained and sensitive individuals as an aura around a person. This emanation is thought to be especially strong around certain centres called chakras (the term comes from India, where this energy is called 'prana').

Bio-energy can also, it appears, be registered on a photograph. A Soviet husband-and-wife research team, Semjon and Valentina Kirlian, discovered that radiation and light phenomena around objects placed in the electrical field of a high-frequency current can be captured on photographic paper. The patterns vary according to health and mental state. One can, for example, see changes around a healer's hands while he/she works.

Bio-energy is one of the factors behind so-called parapsychological phenomena such as clairvoyance, thought-transference, pre- and postcognition (the ability to see into the future and the past), telekinesis (the ability to move or effect changes in objects without touching them) and psychic healing.

Sensitives are thus people who can *consciously* control, direct and utilize bio-energy. We all use and are affected by bio-energy in our daily lives, but without being aware of it.

In Russia, traditional folk-knowledge in this area seems

to have survived to a much greater degree than is the case in Western Europe. The reasons for this are undoubtedly numerous.

This vast land was well into modern times a third-world country with few doctors, where boards of health and similar institutions had difficulties in making their presence felt. The Orthodox Church is also more open to popular mysticism and irrationality than the Catholic and Protestant Churches. The fact that much of this was forced underground after 1917 does not necessarily imply that it has grown weaker.

In the Soviet Union, state and scientific institutions have also taken great interest in the investigation of paranormal phenomena. For example, the possibility of transmitting messages over long distances by thought-transference has been studied. Attempts have also been made to find practical applications within, for example, agriculture. In one case crops were increased by allowing sensitives to exert an influence upon the sowing. In the West, there are speculations as to whether military motives lie behind the Soviet interest in parapsychology.

In a number of Soviet hospitals, sensitives work as healers, side by side with doctors, under scientific control and evaluation.

The theoretical point of departure for their work is that disease is above all caused by disturbances in the energy flow. The physical body is then weakened and left more open to bacterial and viral attack and to other destructive processes. Sensitives can consciously transmit their own bio-energy to the patient and cleanse the biofield of disturbing elements as well as find out what is causing the disturbance. All of this is necessary as a background to understanding certain of Igor's arguments.

He speaks for example of the poor environment in a maternity hospital, where the biofields of many tense people intrude upon and disturb one another, constituting a much

65

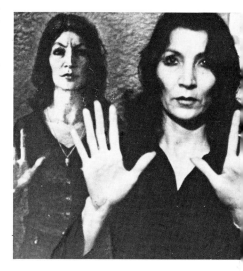

Georgiskan Djuna Davitashvily is a Soviet healer who has also attracted attention in the West. On Swedish television, she has demonstrated how she can, at some distance from the patient's body, 'feel' diseases or injuries with her hands in the form of changes in the patient's biofield. She can also use her hands to transmit her own bioenergy to the patient. She says of her own work: 'I believe that I am doing what Chinese acupuncturists have done for centuries: I activate the body's own defence mechanisms so that the patient can fight his own disease. In the future, when we know more about bioenergy and its properties, we will also be able to work preventatively, so that illness need never arise.'

greater health risk than the presence of bacteria. He is also convinced that sensitives not only can sense whether something is going wrong with mother or child, they can also, with their powers, prevent it from happening.

Igor thus assumes in his work that telepathic contact exists, and is especially strong between mother and child. His belief that the unborn child is affected by what its mother thinks, feels and experiences is the basis for his training of the expectant mother.

He is also referring to this telepathic contact when he emphasizes the danger involved in allowing strangers to be present during the baby's water training. They transmit their anxiety to the baby who can suffer severe stress.

A baby is especially sensitive and vulnerable because it has a completely open biofield. It soaks up impressions like a sponge. (Perhaps people had an inkling of this in the past, when there were countless rules and customs aimed at protecting the child from evil powers during the period immediately following birth.)

This point cannot be over-emphasized. The most dangerous part of the entire water-training process is the horror most people feel when they see a newborn floundering, apparently helpless, in the water. Since water, especially seawater, accumulates and facilitates the transmission of bio-energy, the effect on the child is especially powerful.

'We didn't take this problem into consideration in the beginning,' says Igor. 'But twenty years ago, when we first began teaching newborns to swim, we occasionally ran into unexpected difficulties. At times we were unable to complete the experiments because the children had violently negative reactions which we could not explain. After a series of experiments with animals, however, we began to track down the problem. We collected numerous pieces of evidence pointing to influence from the mother.

When we were teaching kittens to swim, they would occasionally show signs of stress although the situation ought not to have been experienced as particularly threatening. These were times when the mother was present. She was terribly shocked by our actions and her fear immediately spread to her offspring.

When a she-beaver was allowed to take over the kittens' care, however, they showed a great aptitude for swimming. They could stay in the water for several hours at a stretch and hold their breaths for up to five minutes.

This explains all the unsuccessful attempts at baby-swimming made by untrained parents. Understanding and willpower alone are not sufficient for the control of one's biofield. It is influenced to a great degree by subconscious phenomena such as our instinctive fear of water.

Suggestion can occasionally be of help in such cases. A much more reliable method, however, is the training-program I've worked out for parents.'

We come to that now.

7 'The baby's experience of

water begins with the mother'

'If one wants to give one's child the chance to become a real "waterbaby", it is not sufficient to start at birth. The mother must begin during pregnancy,' says Igor.

'What the mother does – how she thinks, behaves and reacts – influences the baby even during the early foetal stages. "Sensitives" have been able to trace a child's psychological problems to frightening experiences the mother has had during pregnancy, and they have also been able to free the child from these problems.

We found more tangible evidence of the way in which the mother's behaviour during pregnancy affects the unborn child when we studied children of professional swimmers who continued their training during pregnancy. Even at birth, these children had much more marked swimming reflexes than other babies. They used actual swimming strokes.

The women who come to me because they want to give birth underwater have made a choice. They believe in an idea, they are fighting for a cause. This positive attitude is essential to the success of the training. Even in the future when underwater birth will, hopefully, be more widely

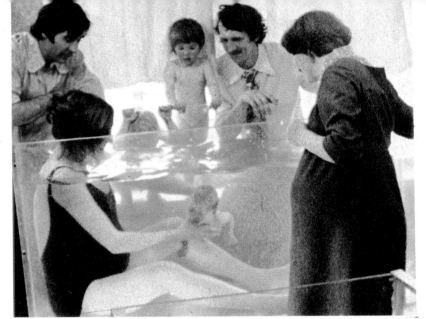

The baby's adaptation to water is actually established before birth; it is thus important for the expectant mother to spend a great deal of time in the water, according to Igor Tjarkovsky. It is also important for the parents to see and meet other parents who are water-training their children under Igor's supervision.

accepted, it will be important for the woman to take a stand, to invest time and effort in careful preparation.

Since the child's adaptation to water is established long before birth, it is important for the mother to spend as much time as possible in the water during pregnancy. She should swim a great deal.

It is also a good idea for the woman to practise swimming, diving and even eating underwater, sucking on a baby bottle, perhaps picking up bits of food from the bottom. Seeing a child suck on a bottle or eat underwater, whether in real life or in a photograph, is not nearly as convincing or effective as doing it oneself.

It is not only a question of physical training, but also of psychological training. It is therefore essential for the expectant mother to be present while other parents are water-training their babies. She must see for herself how babies enjoy being in water, how good it is for them and how safe it can be if one follows certain rules. She must try to empathize with the children's enjoyment; to see, and truly realize, that it is possible. Not dangerous – just fun.

Naturally, it is a good idea for her to meet other parents who have delivered and trained their children in water and talk to them about their experiences.

The mass media can also play an important role. Reading articles or seeing television programmes about underwater birth and the water-training of newborns can be very helpful to the mother. This type of publicity, so long as it is matter-of-fact and objective, can do much to help eliminate people's instinctive fear of water.

This training must be carried out with a firm hand,' says Igor. 'One can't help the woman to overcome her prejudices and her deep-rooted fear of water simply by telling her that these prejudices and fears are unfounded. Much more is needed to convince her, to combat an attitude inherited through millions of years.

All of this preparation is directed towards the great occasion. The delivery. At last the day has come.

Everything is ready. The delivery room is prepared with a large glass-walled tank of warm water which must accommodate not only the mother but also the midwife, the male midwife and the father.

The father provides practical help and reassurance for the mother and he contributes his energy. The father is often much more exhausted by the delivery than the mother.

The tank must be deep enough to allow observers to dive down properly. The more they can stay underwater the better.

Stillness and calm reign in the room. The light is subdued, disturbing impressions from the surroundings screened off. It is important that all those present are in accord with what is about to take place. Negative reactions such as anxiety or doubt are transmitted to mother and child and can have a dangerous influence upon them.

Perhaps, as we have already mentioned, a "sensitive" is present in the delivery room. A surgeon and a paediatrician are informed and ready to intervene should the necessity arise. During the underwater births which have taken place up to now, they have very rarely been called on. The warm water in the tank acts as an effective pain-reliever. Moreover, energy consumption decreases in water. Both mother and baby thus have more strength to cope with the delivery and the decisive last moments.

Since sensations of pain are reduced, the mother can also concentrate on controlling her own movements and working with her body in the most effective way. Her weightlessness in water enables her easily to take on any position which feels suitable.

Lying on one's back, which is the "normal" position in our hospitals, is probably the worst, partly because it is more difficult to push the baby out during the final stage of the delivery and partly because the body is weaker in this position. The woman not only feels helpless and paralyzed, but experiments have also shown that lying on one's back weakens the organism. In the water, the mother can adopt all sorts of positions. All fours often proves suitable, as well as contorted, asymmetrical positions. During certain stages, the path of the foetus is actually asymmetrical, spiralling.

The delivery assistants dive down, observe the proceedings and help out underwater if necessary.

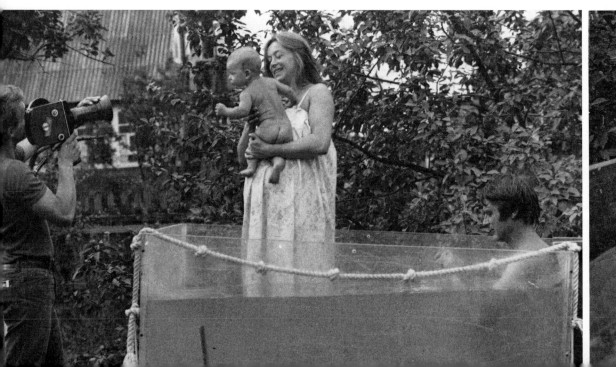
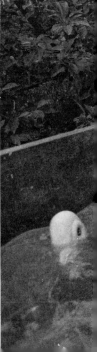

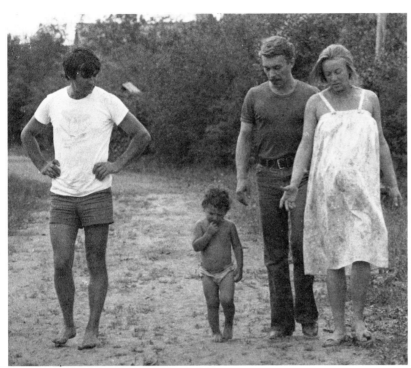

The actress Margarita Tereshkova is one mother who has water-trained her child. She has, among other things, worked in the films of Soviet director Andre Tarkovsky. When Margarita was expecting her second child, she put herself through a regular, intensive water-training programme under Igor's guidance. Although she didn't deliver under water (doctors advised against it since she was over 40 at the time) she began water-training her son immediately after delivery.

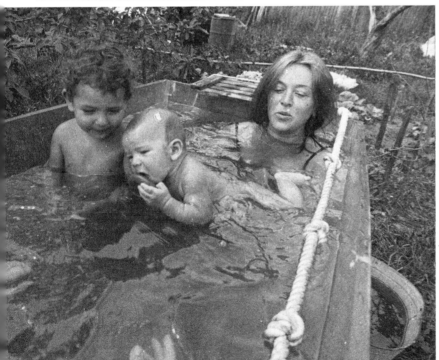

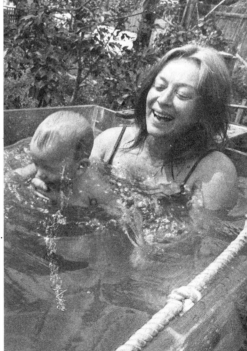

For the baby, emergence from the mother is not the dramatic event of a normal delivery. It doesn't come out into a cold world where the force of gravity strikes like the blow from a club. One warm, body-supporting liquid is exchanged for another. The first breath, for many of us forced out with a smack, is not something which must occur in this present, stressful moment when all is happening at once: light, gravity, lifting up, cutting the cord.

A newborn baby can endure a lack of oxygen far better than an adult, whose lungs are of course in full operation. The umbilical cord also functions for several minutes after birth.

The mother can therefore slowly, gently, catch up her child in the water and bring it to her breast. Perhaps it will immediately find a nipple to suck on. In any case it will be resting securely in the same element and the same energy-field in which it has lived for the last nine months.

Gently, carefully, when the time feels right, the mother can raise herself slightly out of the water. The baby feels the air against its face while its body is still in the water. It can draw an experimental first breath. The transition to breathing air, to a life on dry land, takes place slowly and softly.

Cutting the cord can also wait.

This is the best possible start for the child, and the longer its existence in water can continue uninterrupted the better,' says Igor. 'It is never too late to begin water-training, but even a week after delivery much has been lost.'

The delivery has begun. The woman entered the tank as soon as the first pains started.

74

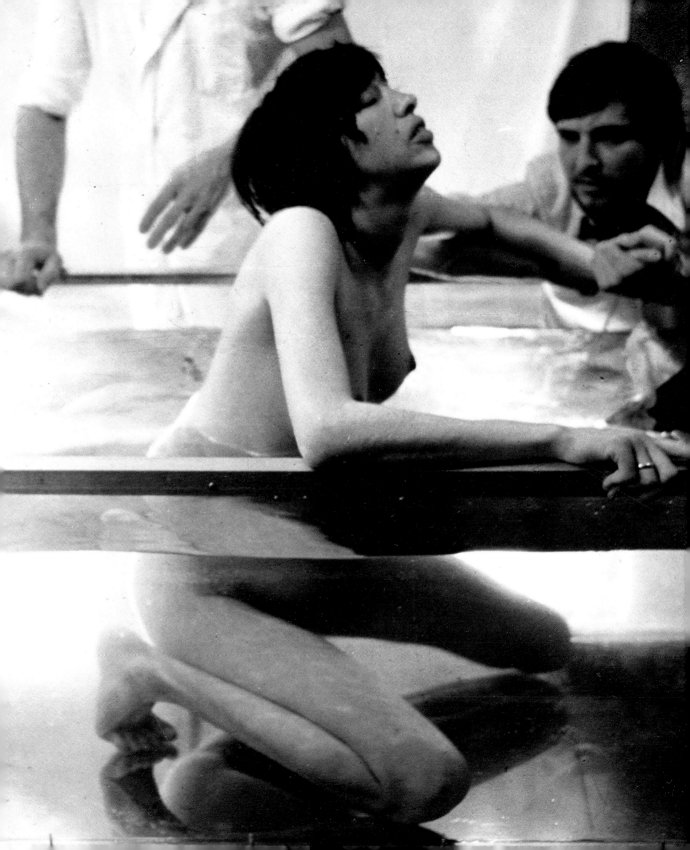

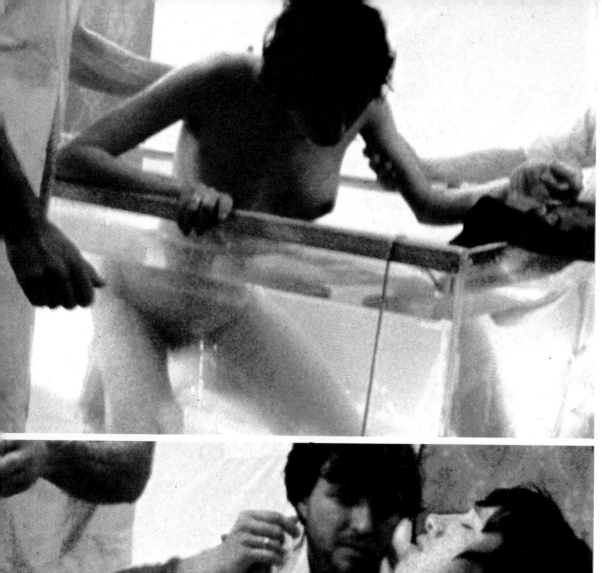
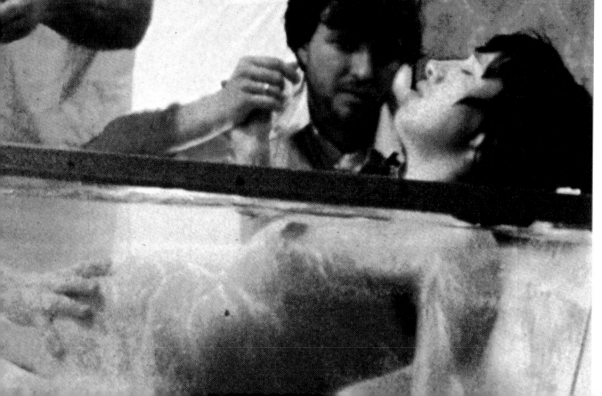

Here we see a young family bring its first child into the world – underwater. These are fantastic photographs of a fascinating process, but in one respect they do not do full justice to what is happening here. For the photographer's sake, the delivery room is brightly lit by strong lamps; a great deal of the intense yet peaceful atmosphere of an underwater delivery is thus lost. An underwater delivery is a real team effort. The unusually well-prepared parents know exactly what to expect and receive intensive guidance from Igor and his assistants. The warm water eases the pain and enables the woman easily to take on any position which feels right at the moment; on her back, on her side or kneeling. Her husband is constantly by her side, resisting her pulling movements or simply holding her hand at difficult moments.

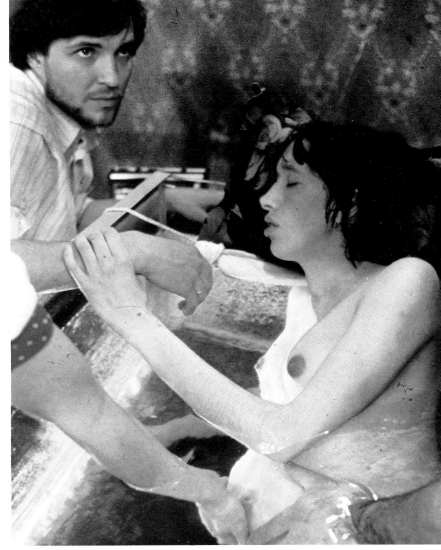

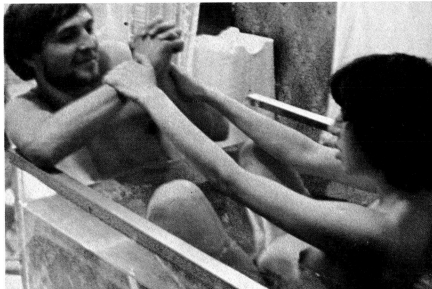

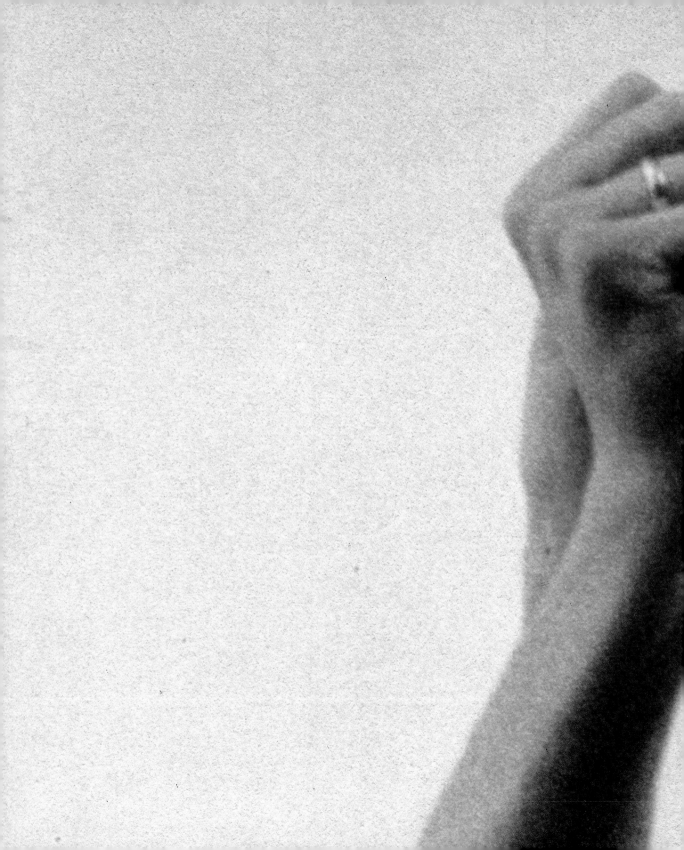

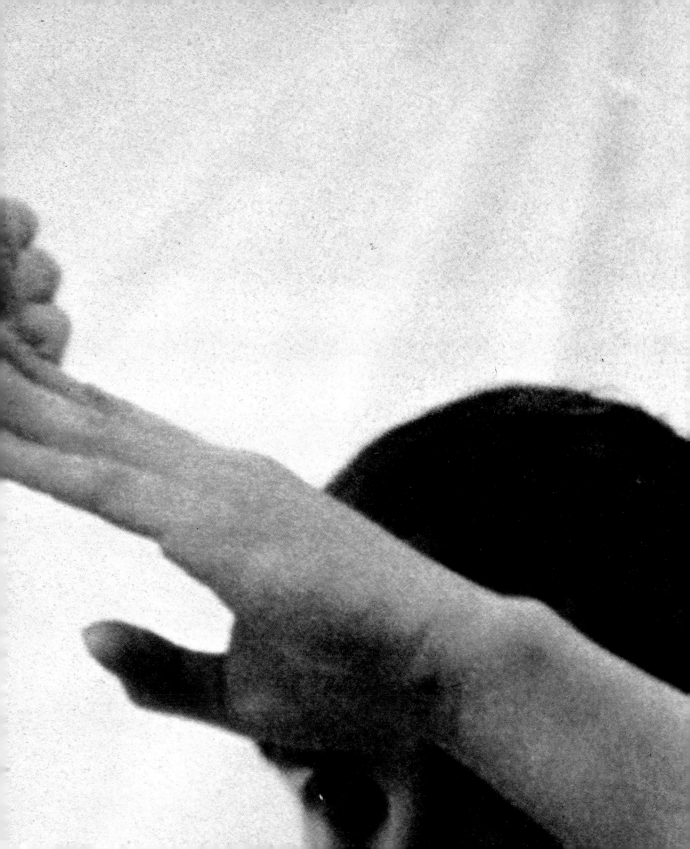

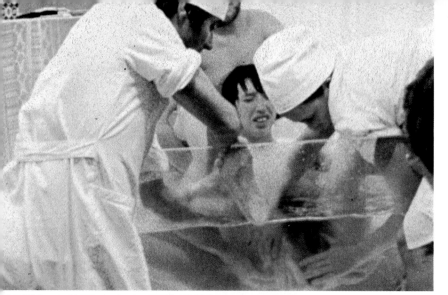

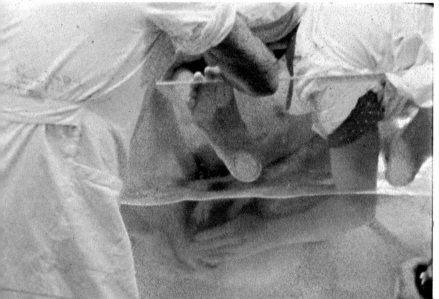

Then comes the final phase – the actual delivery. The baby's dark head pokes out of the opening. The midwife pulls gently so that the next time the woman bears down, the baby pops out. Though the baby makes contact with the outside world, it is still a familiar place, the weightless world of water. The infant is looked after carefully, at first under the water's surface. After a short while the mother lifts it up unhurriedly, gently, carefully, to meet the air and the force of gravity.

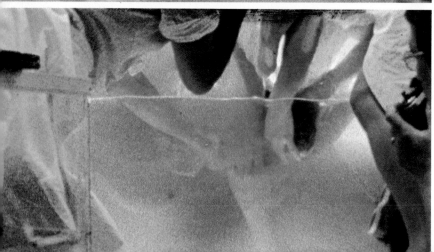

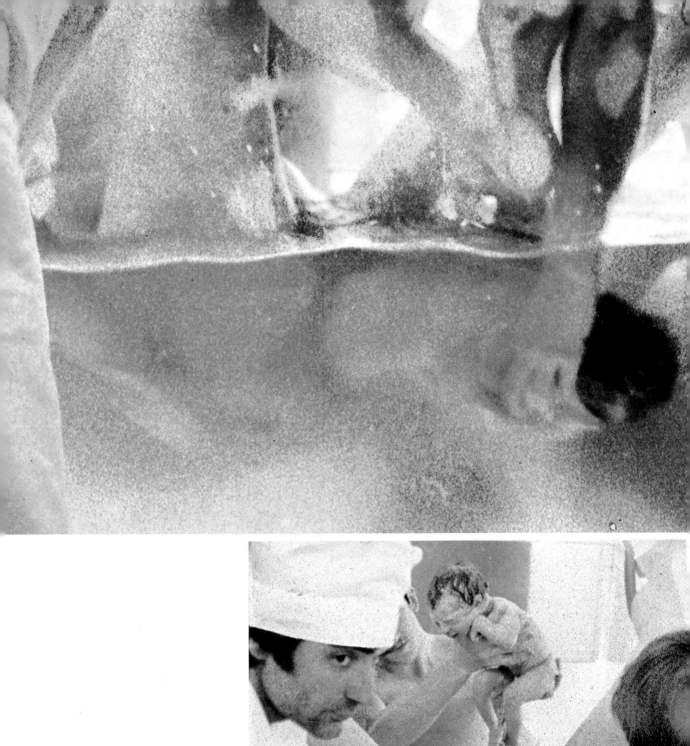
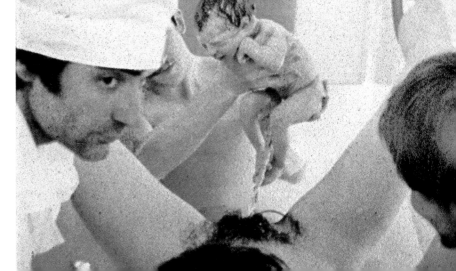

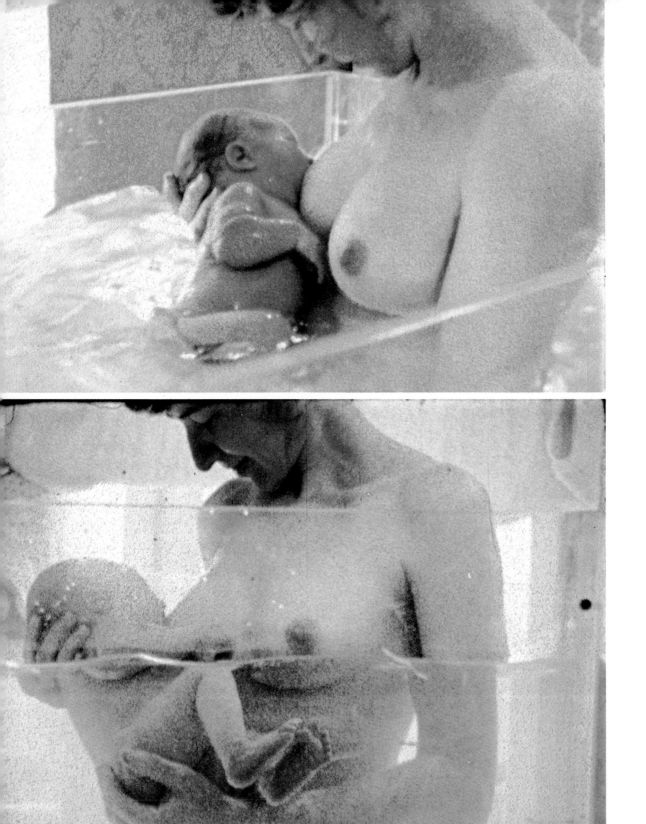

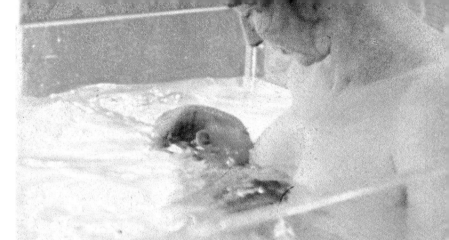

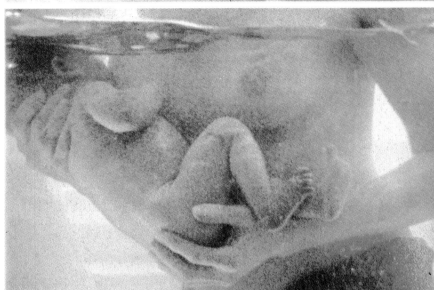

It may look hazardous, but underwater nursing increases enjoyment of food and body contact. Naturally, the mother must lift the baby out of the water from time to time to give it air. Under experienced guidance, she soon relaxes into a calm rhythm, adapted to the needs of the child.

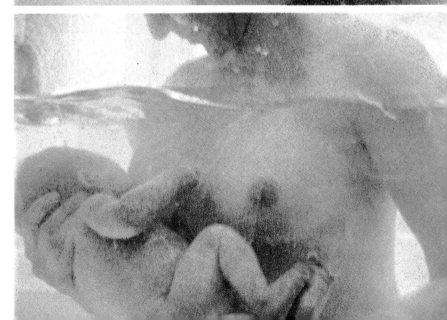

8   'Let experience

speak for itself'

So much can be said and written about the theory of underwater birth and water-training. But what have they been like for those who have experienced them personally? We've chosen three parents who describe their experiences.

These are not a set of how-to instructions. Work in this area cannot be done according to a formula, and individual reactions are paramount. Individual experiences can never be regarded as universal, but similarities can certainly be seen and sensed.

Case history 1

'Did your wife deliver in water or did you begin with water-training?'

'No, she had a normal delivery. As a matter of fact, we weren't even aware that the possibility for underwater birth existed. We'd only heard that Doctor Tjarkovsky trained newborns in water, and we thought it sounded fantastic.'

'How did you start with this training?'

'We invited Dr. Tjarkovsky to our home when our daughter was ten weeks old. He brought an extremely heavy satchel with him, I remember, filled with photographs and newspaper clippings and other papers. We'd really only intended to have a chat with him, get an idea of what the whole thing was about, find out how to begin and so forth.

We talked and looked at photographs, but then Dr. Tjarkovsky said that he could give us a practical example right on the spot. We hadn't expected this, but we couldn't really back out.'

'Tell me – what did he do then?'

'Well, you could say that he started with gymnastics. He grasped our daughter by the leg and started to swing her around. We thought it seemed unusual, to say the least, but the interesting thing was that she obviously seemed to be enjoying the treatment.

I understood then, for the first time, that our ideas about what feels good or bad do not necessarily apply to children. This insight helped us overcome our feelings of unease later on, when we started water-training our daughter on our own.

Dr. Tjarkovsky then asked us to fill the bathtub with water. We filled it with 99°F water but he said this was too warm. We added cold water until the temperature was down to about 86°F.

When he put our daughter in the water she started screaming. She'd never liked being washed. But Dr. Tjarkovsky started playing with her and she soon stopped.

He said that before you dip a child under the surface of the water, you must say some key words which the child will gradually learn to associate with being dipped. This helps the child learn to hold its breath. The key words can be "one-two-*three*" or "oh hey-oh-*ho*" or simply "oh-*now*". You must say them more loudly and clearly than anything else you say while the child is in the water.

It is also important to pay close attention to when the baby breathes in. You should dip it immediately afterwards. It will then breathe out underwater, which helps prevent it from swallowing water. Gradually, he said, the child acquires a breathing rhythm.

Well, after he had explained all this to us, he grasped our daughter under the arms and dipped her under the water.'

'How did she – and you – react?'

'When she came up she started screaming, but not really very much. Dr. Tjarkovsky didn't let her continue for long but dipped her under the water again.

He explained to us afterwards that the baby screams as it breathes out and that it should be dipped again *before* it starts to scream. Hearing its own scream frightens and overexcites the baby.

Our own reactions? I must admit that they were extremely negative. I got spasms all over my body and my wife was as white as a sheet. Dr. Tjarkovsky said that if he hadn't been there to counterbalance our reactions they would have had an extremely dangerous and negative effect upon our daughter.'

'What happened next?'

'As far as I recall, Dr. Tjarkovsky dipped our daughter into the water five or six more times. Then he took her out of the water. We wanted to wrap her up warmly right away, but Dr. Tjarkovsky said that we must not do this.

He instructed us to lay her on the bed without even drying her off and to spread a thin cotton blanket over her. We had to place her on her stomach. This was absolutely necessary, he said. The baby must not lie on its back after water-training because it can throw up water and choke on it. Quite soon she fell asleep.'

'You say that your first reaction was negative. How did you overcome these negative feelings?'

'We actually did this that very same evening after Dr. Tjarkovsky had left. When we were alone we sat down by our daughter's bed.

We were terribly nervous and just sat gazing at her, certain that at any moment we would notice some terrible damage inflicted upon her by the experience she'd been through.

But she slept on as peacefully as anything. I've never seen anyone sleep so peacefully. Babies are always so sweet and touching when they're asleep and it wasn't the first time we'd seen something like it (we have an older daughter too). But there was something very special about her this evening which made us believe that she had experienced something which we ourselves would never be able to experience or even imagine.

"Isn't she just like an angel?" said my wife and it really was true. It's impossible to describe. Perhaps one of the great Renaissance painters could have captured her expression.

Then, in the space of a moment, all our anxiety disappeared. We just sat there, admiring her. It was an unforgettable experience for us both.

After about two hours she woke up and my wife breast-fed her. Then she slept again as usual, right through to morning.'

Case history 2

'How old was your son when you first began water-training him?'

'He was three weeks old.'

'Did Dr. Tjarkovsky say that this was a good age to start?'

'Yes, he said that it was pretty good. As far as I know, the earlier you start the better.'

'At first you worked under his guidance, if I've understood correctly. When did you begin training your son on your own?'

'We'd never done anything like this before, of course – we'd only seen newborns in water on film, so Dr. Tjarkovsky said we should be very cautious. In the beginning the most important thing was not to be afraid when we saw our son in the water. Therefore, I was to start by simply playing with him in the bathtub – no dipping allowed. Sometimes I would even get into the tub with him myself and feed him there. So water became associated in his mind with the pleasure of receiving food.

When I felt that we both were ready, I began doing dipping exercises with him, extremely simple ones at first. For example, I pressed his face against my breast to keep water from getting into him and let him sink down with me under the surface of the water. After a time, we began doing the exercises which Dr. Tjarkovsky had shown us.'

'Did your son enjoy all this?'

'No, not in the beginning. But he became inured to it after a while. Besides, he had so much else to do! He no longer minded the water-training, not because it made him frightened or nauseous, but because it kept him from his play. I therefore tried to arrange things so that he could be underwater and play at the same time. I placed non-floatable toys on the bottom of the tub so he would have to dive down to get them. I scattered cranberries on the bottom and he would swim underwater until he'd picked them all up.'

'Did you meet Dr. Tjarkovsky again?'

'Yes. After about a month, we went to see him again. I showed him what I was doing with my son and he said that I could continue on my own. He "examined" my husband too.'

Comment. It is very important that parents who wish to water-train their babies should talk to an expert first, preferably one who is 'sensitive'. Eventually, perhaps, normal parents with extensive experience of water-training will be able to 'examine' other parents.

'Passing' this exam, however, does not qualify parents to water-train other people's babies. A strong telepathic contact generally exists between parents and children, which is why parents often sense the right thing to do with their baby in critical situations. Parents do not have this type of contact with other people's children, which is why an uneducated trainer can, for example, fail to notice that a child is too tired to continue training.

Hopefully, however, the number of people sufficiently qualified to work with other people's children will increase in the future.

'Did you use any objects or pieces of equipment during training?'

'A few very simple ones. Dr. Tjarkovsky constructed most of them himself, but I know that nowadays many people invent their own equipment to use during water-training.

We had, among other things, a specially-constructed baby bottle with a curved nipple for our son to suck on underwater. This bottle could also be fastened on to the bottom of the tub or pool so that the baby had to dive for it.

90

We used a special ladder in the pool – even toddlers could climb up out of the water on it.

Though all of these objects are simple, the problem is that one nearly always has to build them oneself. There are no manufacturers of such accessories.'

'Would you say that your son is different from other children and if so, in what way?'

'Oh, absolutely. Both physically and psychologically. During his first year I took him for regular check-ups at the children's health clinic, where I was able to compare him with other children of the same age. Of course I know that every mother thinks that her own child is the best in the world, but my son really did seem much more advanced in many ways than other children, even older ones.

First of all, he was incredibly active, or rather other children seemed to me incredibly passive. When my son was only a month old he could hold his head steady. At three months he could sit, at seven months he could walk. He lost interest quite early in simple toys such as rattles and began leafing through books instead. He would sit looking at the pictures for hours.

I can state with absolute assurance that water-training was extremely beneficial for him.'

'How old is he now?'

'He's just turned five.'

'Do you still take him swimming?'

'Yes, of course. The trips to and from the pool take a lot of time and energy, but I feel it would be awfully stupid to stop now.'

Case history 3

'Were you afraid to deliver underwater?'

'I was afraid to deliver at all! Doing it in water seemed less awful than the usual way. Besides, I felt great trust in Dr. Tjarkovsky and in the sensitives who were assisting him.'

'Did you use a tank?'

'Yes.'

'When did you get into it?'

'As soon as the pains began.'

'And you stayed in it the entire time?'

'No, I got out once in a while.'

'What happened the first time you got into the water?'

'The pains got weaker and there were longer intervals between them. I felt much less frightened. In fact, I almost felt high in some way. I think I sang.

Later, when the pains got stronger again, I wanted to get back into the water. We had a real midwife with us, however – she'd promised to help out although she didn't approve of underwater deliveries, and she didn't like my spending so much time in the tank. She said that if the water eased the pain and lengthened the intervals between pains, it also meant that the delivery would take longer. She wasn't sure I could handle it if the delivery lasted the whole night.

But Dr. Tjarkovsky let me stay in the water as long as I wanted. I probably saved a lot of energy that way and it came in useful later on when I had to push the baby out.'

'So you believe, generally speaking, that it was good to spend so much time in the water?'

'I think the entire first stage of the delivery was significantly less painful and exhausting than it might have been "on land". I was also able to spread out my energy consumption more evenly. I didn't tire myself out.'

'Did you try to sleep in the water?'

'Yes, but the water was quite warm and that made it hard to breathe. We hadn't thought of bringing something for me to lean against in the water, either.'

'How long did the final stage of the delivery last?'

'A little over half an hour.'

'Weren't you afraid that the baby would get an infection?'

'As far as I understand, the sensitives saw to it that this would not happen.'

'What happened when the baby came out?'

'My husband cut the umbilical cord.'

'Why did he do that?'

'Sensitives believe that if the father does this in the water, he creates a real bond between himself and the child. I think this is even included as a rite in certain religions.'

'What happened next?'

'I think everybody drank champagne. Except the baby, of course.'

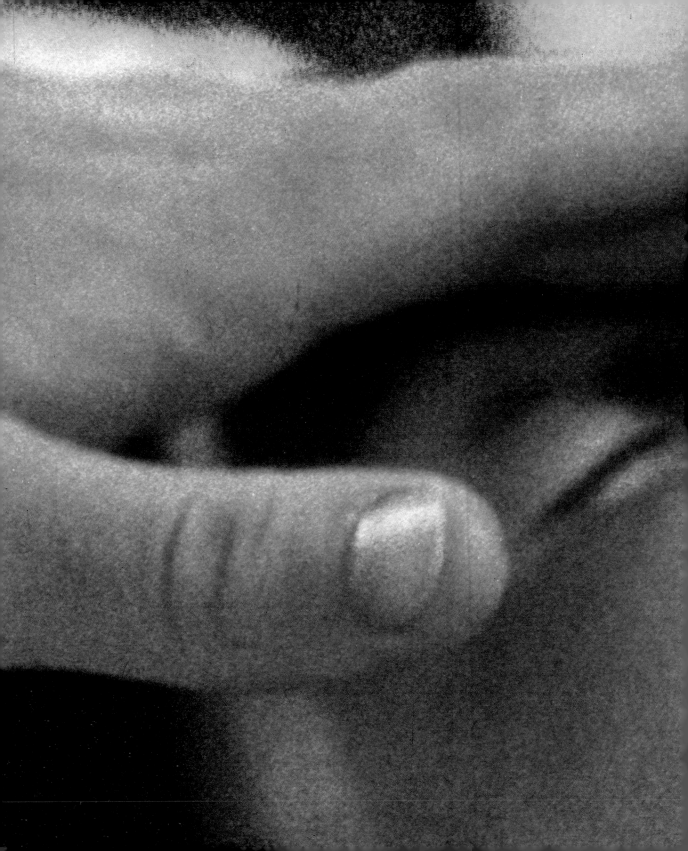

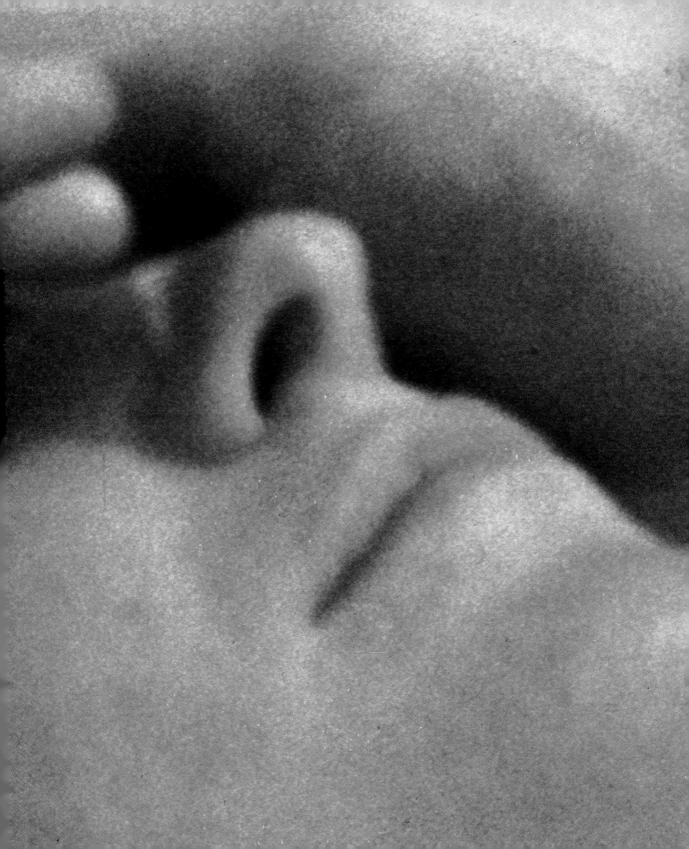

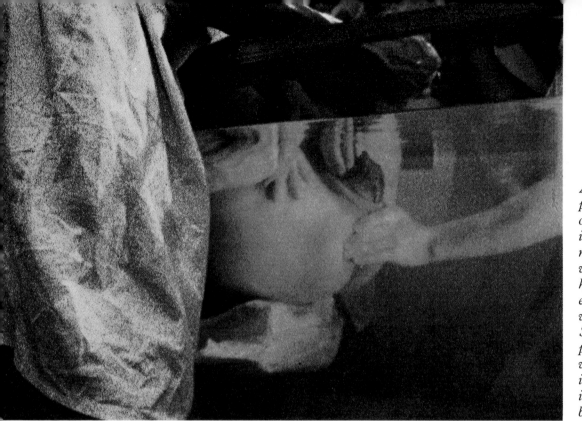

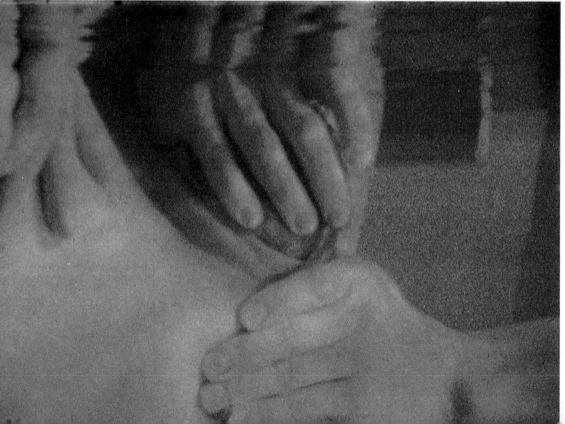

A series of photographs of the awe-inspiring moment when a new human being enters the world. Slowly, it pushes its way out. It is helped out into the body-temperature water, which is clear until a few drops of blood colour it bronze. An eternity and an instant. The newborn child is met by a large, firm hand, still under the surface of the water.

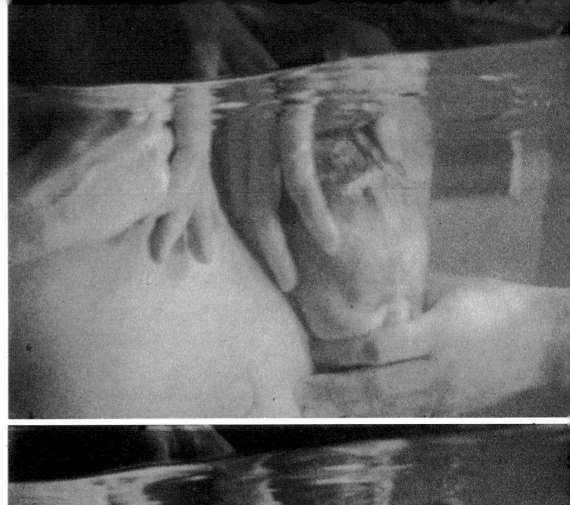

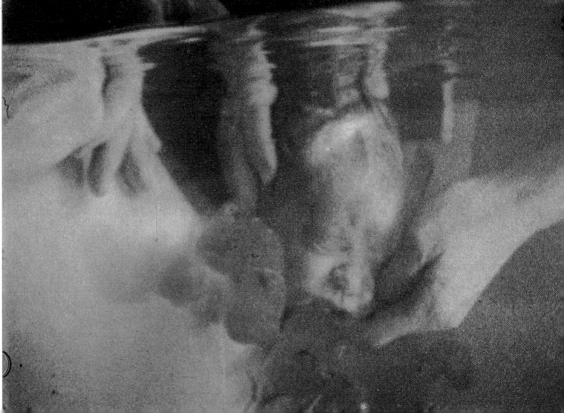

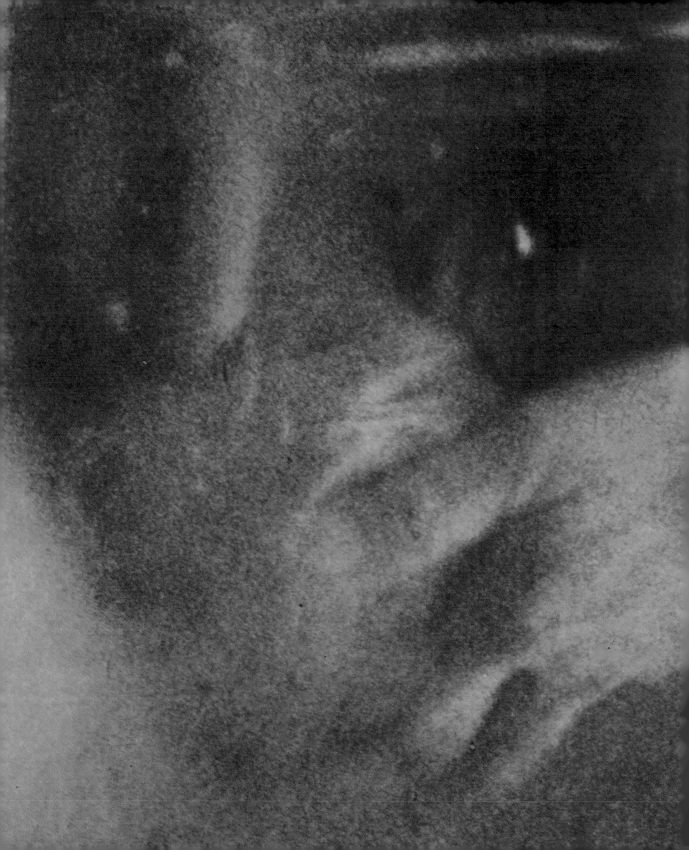

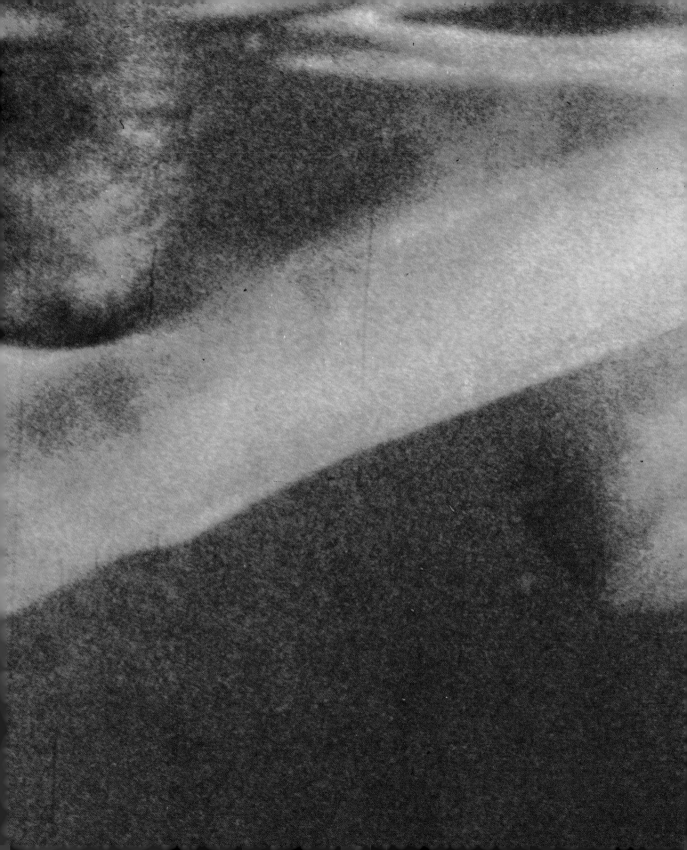

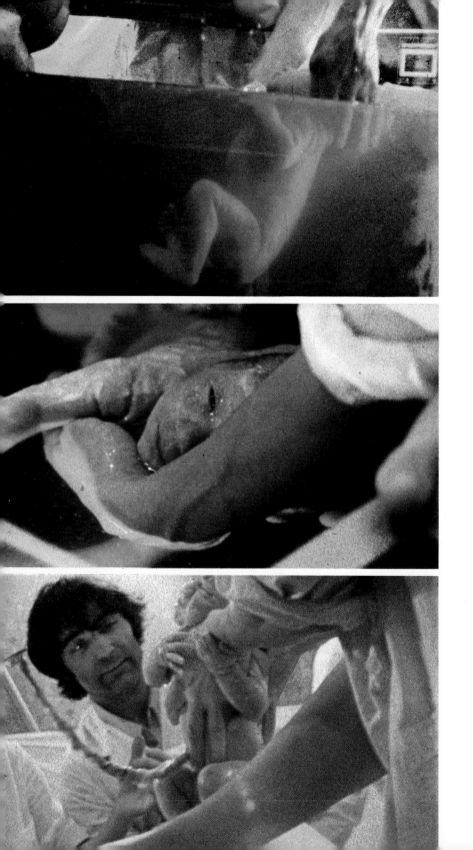

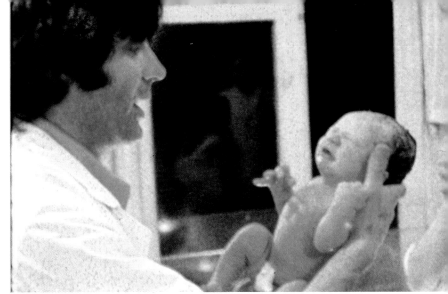

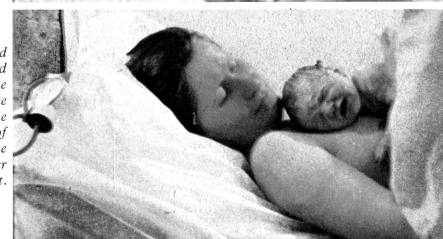

The newborn is lifted carefully out of the water and Igor takes over to cut the umbilical cord and examine the infant. Once out of the water, in the new element of air, it's nice to lie on the mother's body, resting on her soft breast.

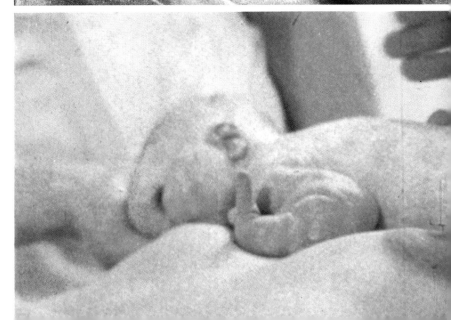

9   Questions for

Tjarkovsky Igor

'Igor, isn't there an enormous risk of infection when a woman delivers underwater?'

'Not at all. This has not been a problem for us. Infections are much more a result of disturbances in the biofield than of the presence of bacteria.

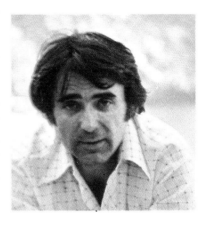

The risk of infection is much greater in the stress-filled environment of a maternity ward or hospital, where the biofields of many tense people collide. The calm, relaxed environment of an underwater birth provides far superior preconditions for an infection-free delivery. There is no risk involved in the husband being in the water with his wife, either, since they live together so intimately that they share the same bacterial flora. A final safety factor is the presence of "sensitives", who cleanse and sterilize the water with their psychic energy.'

'Does it make any difference when one begins the baby's water-training? Doesn't the so-called "diving-reflex" disappear after a certain age?'

'The most important factor is not the physiological reflex itself, but rather the instinctive fear of water created in us by the evolutionary process. It is true that the longer after birth one waits, the stronger this fear becomes.

However, all human beings have the ability to close off the respiratory tract to keep water from entering the lungs. It is this reflex which comes into play when we drink.

Because of this terror of water, however, one must be very gentle and careful when training older babies and children. Proceed gently and playfully. Place orange sections and other good things to eat on the bottom of the pool or tub so that the child will want to bend down and pick them up. Put up pictures on the pool walls so he will have to stay underwater in order to look at them. Let him be in the water along with other, water-trained children – children do imitate one another.

'Is it really healthy to spend so much time in swimming pools? There's so much chlorine in the water.'

'I am personally quite sensitive to chlorine and prefer to wear swimming-goggles. Babies seem to tolerate chlorine better, however, and one seldom notices any problems.

It would be better without chlorine, naturally. Seawater is ideal because it is both clean and has qualities which facilitate psychic contact. An outdoor swimming pool in the fresh air, under the open sky, is naturally also better than a pool in a glassed-in swimming-hall.'

'A little while ago you mentioned how the custom of swaddling babies makes them totally helpless. But in the changing room at the pool I saw several swaddled babies. Why don't you speak to their parents?'

'Ohhh, I'd have to put up posters and banners all over the country, and I don't have the resources. But of course I mention it to them. It's difficult to do anything about it, however. It's not enough if mothers and grandmothers understand. This is more than an ancient custom – the roots go deeper than that. All animals stiffen up, hold still when they're frightened because then the enemies, the hunters, don't notice them. Hunting animals react to movement. I have done experiments with cats and mice which demonstrate this principle. I bound the mice so that they lay perfectly motionless, and the cats totally lost interest in them.

It is a deep-seated instinct which makes a frightened woman stop short and press her child to her breast hard, so that it won't move, and won't scream. To be on the safe side the child is always kept swaddled, motionless, for there has never been a lack of fear in this country.'

'Isn't it dangerous for newborns to swallow a lot of water, and can one be completely certain that they won't get any into their lungs?'

'All babies swallow water, even in the uterus. There are even methods for adding nutrients to the amniotic fluid so that the foetus, by drinking it, can compensate for a deficiently functioning placenta.

Newborns will also swallow water if placed in it. No normal baby, however, will allow water to enter its lungs. An innate reflex sees to this. Even an adult can dive under water, open his mouth, take a gulp and swallow, and he automatically blocks off his windpipe. Animals have this ability as well. Haven't you seen a horse drinking from a lake with half of its head submerged in the water?

Babies born in water can also make free use of their sense of taste, one of our oldest senses. Taste plays little part in the life of an adult. For a child in water, however, taste is one of the most reliable methods of orientation. Even in the dark it can find its way to its mother.'

'Igor, would you say that you have a method for teaching newborns to swim that anybody can use?'

'No, absolutely not, and this is a very important distinction. I want the *ideas* behind my activities to receive the greatest attention, not the activities themselves – the "method".

A method is a list of instructions which one follows in order to achieve a predetermined result. No such instructions for underwater delivery or the water-training of newborns exist. I have, through experience, discovered certain practical solutions. But one must never under-estimate the risks involved in starting on one's own without special preparation, perhaps looking upon the whole thing as a kind of physical training.

It must be repeated over and over again that there are many factors which must be taken into account and considered. There are great risks involved and many opportunities for mishaps to occur if one is not careful.'

'What are the most common causes of mishaps during water-training?'

'Most people would guess that the danger lies in the child swallowing water or getting water into its lungs. But as I've mentioned, newborns automatically close off the windpipe under water. In most cases the problem originates outside the tub or the pool. I'll tell you about a case where I was called to see a little boy who was apparently suffering from a lack of oxygen. What had happened?

The father had trained his son for an hour in the bathtub, then wrapped him up lightly in a blanket and placed him on his stomach. The child had then thrown up some water, as many babies do after water-training. There is nothing dangerous about it. His grandmother saw this, however, and nearly fainted in horror. She snatched the child to her and began to moan and wail. It was at this point that the boy began having difficulties.

I've seen so many examples of how grandmothers have nearly killed their own grandchildren that I feel justified in saying that grandmothers should be kept away during water-training.'

'What about other people, then?'

'Since I am quite convinced that the greatest danger for the baby lies in the reaction of outsiders, I believe that their number should be limited. One or both parents and perhaps an instructor would be ideal.

It's understandable that proud parents want to show off their child to friends and acquaintances when it begins making progress, but they should absolutely not do this. It would mean exposing the child to serious risks.'

'I've seen photographs of babies swimming backstroke. Is this a good method?'

'No, not at all. I strongly advise against it. Perhaps it's a position which suits the swimming teacher.

First of all, it is dangerous for the child. As far back as the 'sixties we realized that lying on one's back weakens the organism and decreases endurance. Furthermore, the windpipe is not closed in this position, as it is when the baby dives underwater. Water can get into the lungs. Parents often feel more secure when they can see the child's face, but this is a false security.

Yes, it really is possible. Igor demonstrates his programme for a hesitant father.

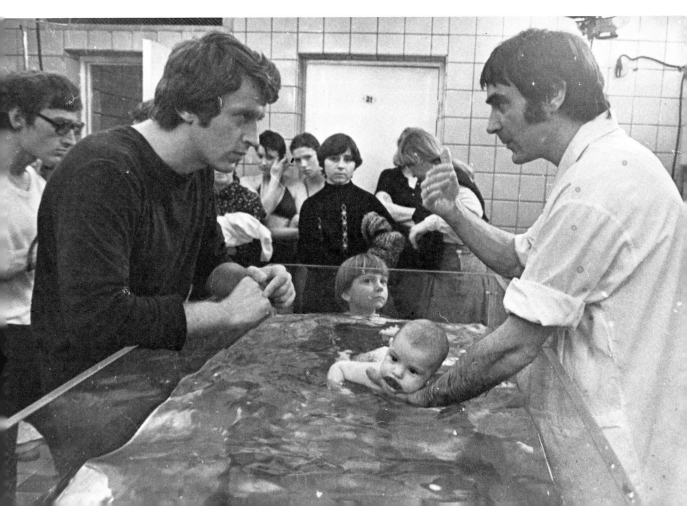

Besides, the baby is helpless in this position. It sees nothing but a white ceiling far above. It cannot investigate the environment. One of the great advantages of water-training is that the baby, even during its first days, can move about freely in three dimensions. It cannot do so while lying on its back.

Unfortunately, it's quite easy to teach babies to paddle around on their backs. Many photographs of this have been shown and it's become quite popular, but I do not recommend it. Lying on its back gets the child nowhere.'

'But isn't it better for the child to swim on its back than not at all?'

'You are operating from a common misconception: you assume that if a child can stay afloat it can swim, and if it can swim it can also adapt to a life in water. This is not at all certain.'

'Igor, when I've spoken to other Russians about your work they haven't always heard of you, but they have been aware of the fact that newborns can be taught to swim. Does this satisfy you?'

'As a matter of fact, no. I'll summarize the situation in this way: In this country, there exists what amounts to a popular movement for teaching babies to swim, officially encouraged by the Ministry of Health. However, the goals and methods have become unbelievably watered-down by a basic misconception: that it's only a question of teaching newborns to swim.

Everything else aside, "baby-swim" in itself is not at all dangerous, as many influential people still maintain. But encouraging early swimming ability is not an effective means of helping a child adapt to a life in water.

Many people have lost sight of the larger goal by focussing on a more limited one – though it certainly is good for babies to swim.

There is another misconception here: many people have received the impression that it is the swimming itself which lies behind the fantastic skills which "my" children can display. But it is above all the practice in diving and holding the breath which is important.

On the other hand, it is also a misunderstanding to assume that these activities are unsuitable for "ordinary" people – that only an elite group should participate in them. They are open to any parent who wants to give his or her child greater opportunities in life than he or she has had.'

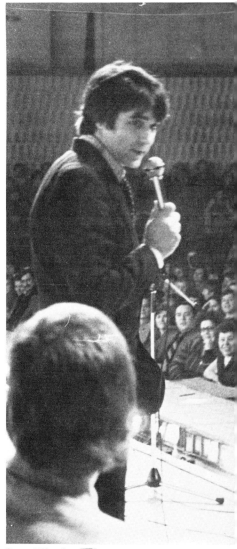

Igor Tjarkovsky has given many lectures in the Soviet Union. He attracts large, interested and inquisitive audiences.

IO 'The baby just becomes

better and better friends
with the water'

'Igor, you say that the principles of water-training cannot be learned by reading a ten-page handbook, and that it is dangerous for uninitiated parents to get started on their own, without a deeper insight into and understanding of what they're doing. But can't you describe a few practical exercises? What are the important elements involved in a training programme?'

'Nursing or feeding the child underwater is extremely important. One should actually begin with this. The best thing, of course, is if the mother herself can breast-feed the child underwater. Those who are for some reason afraid to do this can instead feed the child underwater with a specially-constructed baby bottle with a long nipple.

When nursing underwater, a baby needs less oxygen. We have come to this conclusion after hundreds of experiments, and we have settled on a reliable method for underwater nursing. When the baby needs air it will stop sucking. For the mother, this is the signal to lift up the baby so that its mouth clears the surface of the water for one breath, and then down again. Gradually, the mother becomes familiar with the child's needs and can relax into a rhythm.

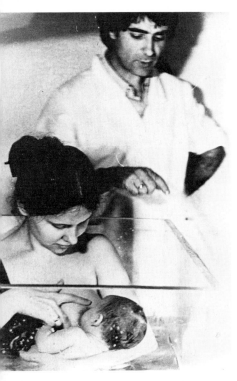

Igor instructs the mother in underwater nursing. When the baby needs air it stops sucking. This is a signal to the mother to lift the baby out of the water. Sucking under water helps the baby learn to hold its breath for several minutes at a time.

Nursing underwater helps the child learn to hold its breath for several minutes at a time, which is one prerequisite for being able to explore the water. Moreover, water becomes associated in the baby's mind with something pleasant.

By the age of two months, the child will generally be able to dive underwater and feed itself. This is important, since it is generally at the age of three months that children develop their fear of water, their perception of it as something terribly dangerous. However, if the child is allowed to experience water as a friendly element right from the beginning, it will not develop this fear and its attitude to water will grow more and more positive.'

'How should one handle babies born in the traditional way, who have spent their first days in the maternity ward and in the cradle at home?'

'I can imagine that many parents in this situation would want to "make up" for lost time. But this isn't possible!

If the child has spent its first few days on "dry land", its body will already have adjusted to this new form of existence. Therefore, one must not water-train such a child too intensively.

This certainly does not mean that one has forfeited all chances. I only want to emphasize that one mustn't try to rush things, but instead proceed gently and cautiously.

Here is a series of exercises suitable for use in a swimming pool or in the bath-tub at home.

Walk just far enough into the pool so that the water reaches your stomach/chest. Lift the child in the air in front of you, toss it up, let go of it for a second and then catch it again.

Most children think this is fun. If you see that the child is smiling or laughing, you can carefully let its feet splash down into the water before catching it. If all is going well, you can grow bolder and bolder and let the child splash deeper and deeper into the water. (This type of game is actually much safer in water than in a normal room with a hard floor – if you should happen to slip, nothing serious can happen since water is so soft to fall into.)

Anyone can invent new variations on this game themselves. You may think that a two-week-old baby wouldn't get much out of such exercises, but they are in fact extremely beneficial. The child gains practice in coordinating its movements, which in turn strengthens muscular and mental skills such as the ability to react. Our comparative experiments with animals have shown that animals who receive this type of simple training can solve various problems more quickly and efficiently.

I've already described the practice of underwater nursing. The rules apply both to breast and bottle feeding. If carried out gently and carefully, underwater nursing can also be very beneficial for babies born in the traditional manner.

Then, of course, there are the basic dipping exercises, which should be done when the baby has begun to display a sense of security in the water. Hold the baby under the armpits, stretch out your arms, say some simple word(s) which the baby will gradually learn to recognize as the signal to hold its breath, then dip the child under the surface of the water. Draw it in towards you, then up again when it reaches your body. Do this over and over again, calmly and rhythmically, letting the child stay underwater for a few seconds at a time. It is best to allow the child one breath only between immersions.

If the child appears tired or starts screaming, it's best to switch to a new exercise or to stop altogether. Screaming is not always a signal that it's time to stop, however – an experienced parent will be able to determine the seriousness of the situation. Perhaps it's just as well to continue calmly, with one breath between immersions.

If the child really grows hysterical, however, you must stop immediately.

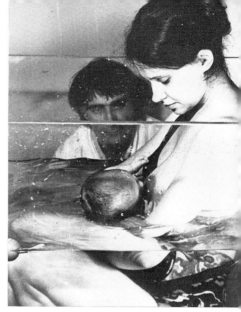
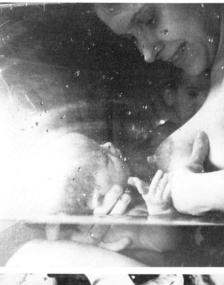
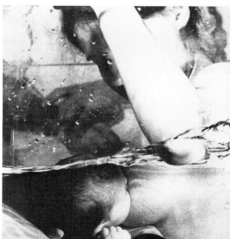

113

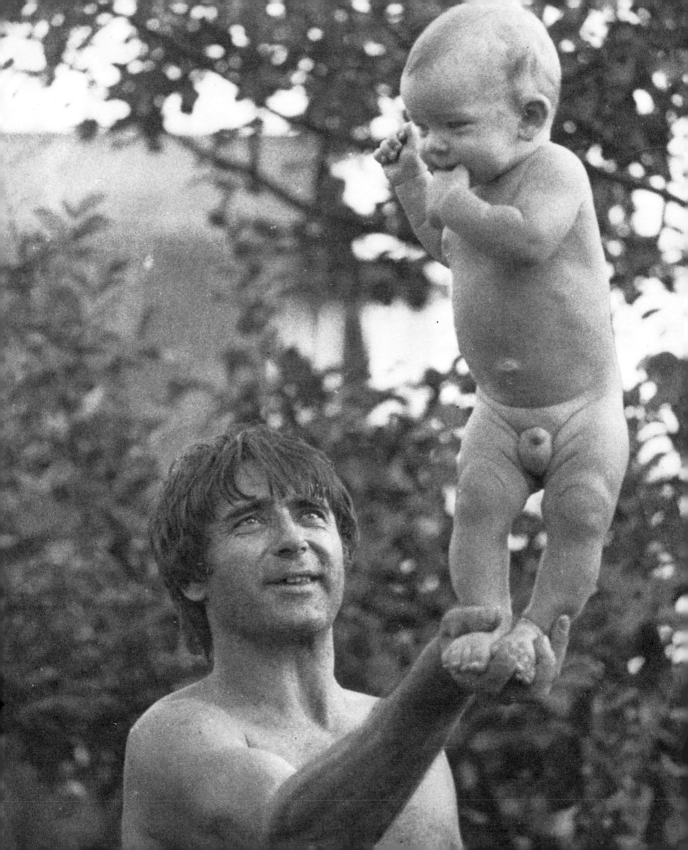

After a while, you can try letting the child *walk* under-water on the bottom of the pool. It is a good idea to use food as stimulation during this exercise. I have constructed a walking-chair which the child can use to support itself while it walks and to which one can fasten a baby bottle.

Most children like walking underwater, but care must be taken that they don't fall and strike themselves as this can be terrifying for them.

These exercises in walking underwater can also help the child learn to walk on land unusually early, around the age of three months. This is a more dynamic method of learning to walk than the usual way, in which the baby first learns to stand and then, gradually, to stumble forward.'

'But is it really healthy for a three-month-old baby to walk?'

'Not according to many experts, and I agree with them as far as normal children are concerned. But well-trained "waterbabies" have muscles like athletes even at this age and for them it can only be positive.

It is precisely this fact – that babies grow strong enough to walk at an incredibly early age – which has convinced many people, including paediatricians, of the very real benefits of water-training. I must admit, however, that I am personally much more interested in the fact that three-month-old babies can swim two or three miles than in the fact that they can walk one hundred yards on land.

In the 'sixties, we worked with a five-year-old boy who would keep swimming as long as one pulled a bottle in front of him. He swam, ate, and slept in the water, and then went right on swimming.

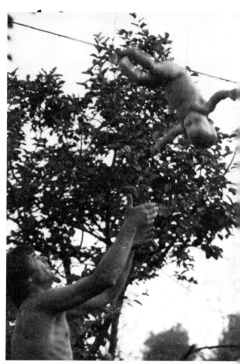

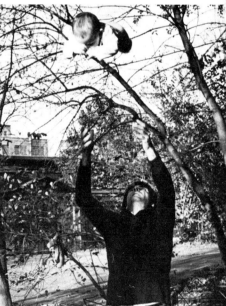

Igor demonstrates how a baby, after several months of water-training, has developed its muscle strength, balance and co-ordination to the point where it can easily balance in the palm of an adult's hand . . .

. . . as well as enjoy somersaults and flips in the air.

115

There is another good exercise to try when the child is a little older. Grasp the child's feet in one hand and lift it up. The other hand can be used to support the child if necessary. The goal here is to have the child stand in the palm of your hand and practise keeping its balance. Don't let go of its feet!

When the child finally falls – perhaps after a few seconds – keep a firm grip on its feet and let it dangle in your hand with its head hanging downwards. It is obvious from their laughter that most youngsters think this is great fun.

Hopping exercises are also good. In the beginning it is best to hold the child's hands and swing or dangle it in the air. Eventually, the child will be able to jump by itself from the side of the pool, but a helping hand may also be needed here.'

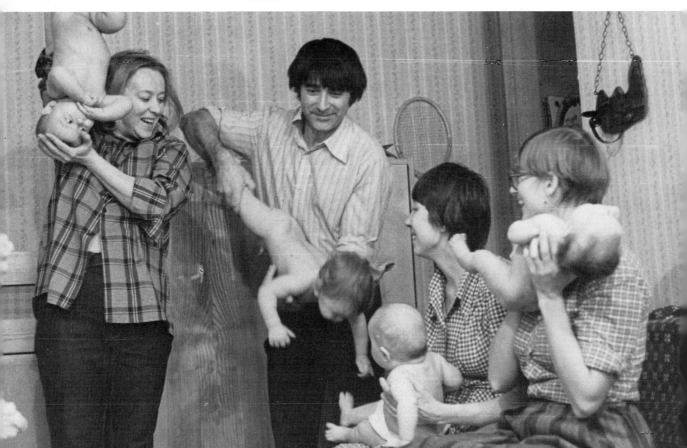

Water-training
makes children
strong and fit.
They naturally
transfer their
abilities to out-of-
water athletics.
There is usually
room in the home
for a few pieces of
athletic apparatus
for the children.
Igor demonstrates
a few exercises for
actress Margarita
Tereshkova.

11   Children swimming –

even with dolphins

One animal which has defied the land animals' taboo against returning to the sea is the dolphin. Its mammal forefathers must have developed on land, then returned to the sea.

Many researchers have taken an intense interest in dolphins. Myths have been spun about them for thousands of years as wise, kind animals who help seafarers and are allied with the divinities of the sea.

There are certain facts which modern researchers can verify. Dolphins have a remarkably high intelligence level. They can communicate with one another in a clear and concentrated language. They are also social beings. They help one another and have in many proven cases come to the aid of drowning people. As most people know, they must also come up to the surface to breathe.

'Dolphins also have a powerful biofield,' says Igor Tjarkovsky. 'As far back as the 'sixties, I wanted to include them in my experiments. For various reasons, however, I wasn't able to do this until just a few years ago.

During the summer of 1979, we (that is, I myself, several researchers from the Institute, female athletes, mothers, women in advanced stages of pregnancy and an assorted

Igor believes that the biofield of the dolphin provides the child with a tremendous sense of security.

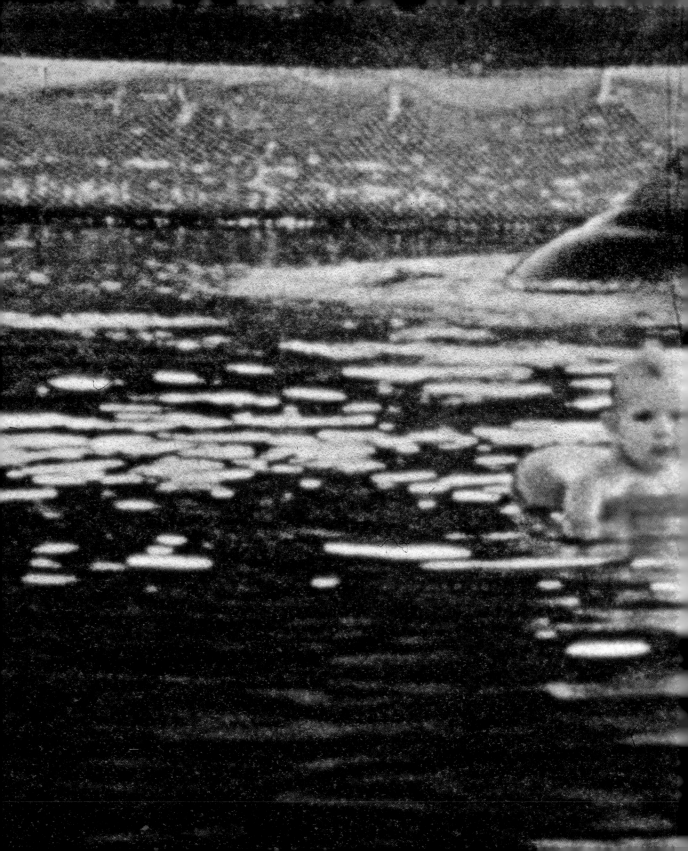

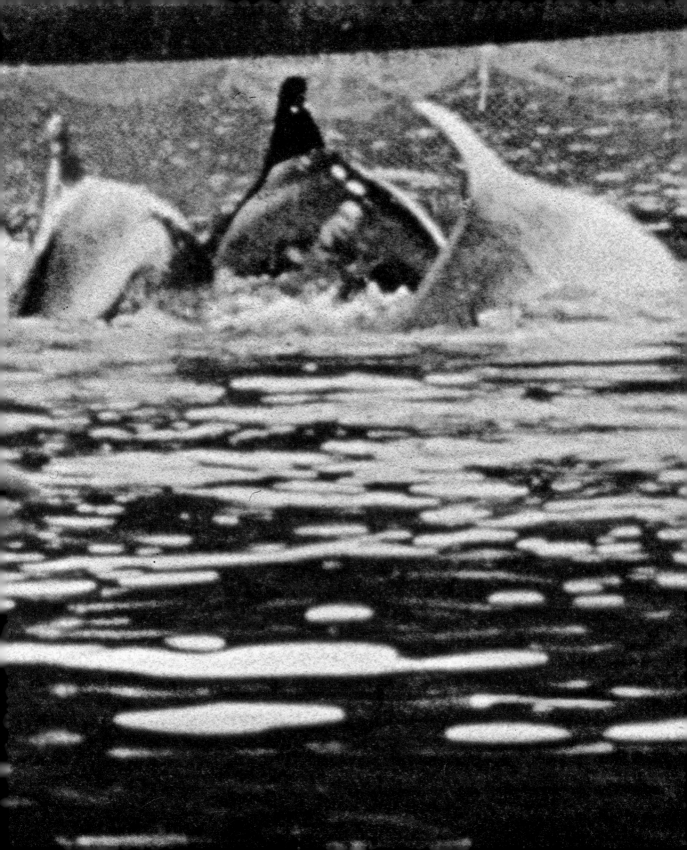

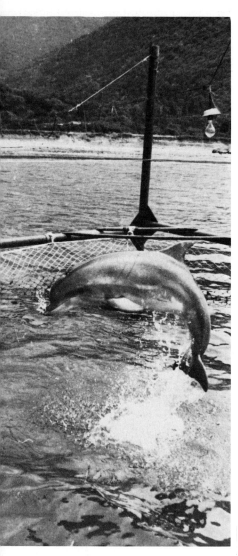

Dolphins are mammals that have returned to the sea. At one time, their ancestors must have been land animals. Dolphins have a highly developed intelligence and some type of language used for advanced communication...

group of children between the ages of eight days and eight years) made an expedition to a dolphin research station by the Black Sea.

We carried out a number of different experiments with the dolphins, some of which we were forced to do at night while the station's regular research staff slept. They didn't like our letting newborns and dolphins loose together because they were afraid to take the risk of the dolphins harming the children.

Absolutely nothing of the kind occurred, however. The dolphins were very gentle with the children. If they came swimming up a little too brusquely, so that the children became frightened, they would immediately slow down, and move at the children's pace.

The dolphins had no objections to anything we did with them, either. We fastened different types of saddles and handles onto their bodies, and they willingly allowed the children to hitch rides on them. Not even the youngest babies were afraid to hold on to the enormous creatures and accompany them when they dived several yards down into the sea after food.

Even more remarkably the dolphins' powerful biofields had a clear effect upon the human beings. The mothers' fear of water vanished. The newborns lay peacefully sleeping in the sea with the dolphins swimming around them.

I especially remember one incident,' says Igor. 'I was working with a one-month-old baby girl underwater, counting the seconds as usual to see when it would be time to swim up. Suddenly, two dolphins came swimming towards me at top speed. At first I thought they were angry. I grew frightened when they shoved me aside and pushed the child up to the surface. But they only wanted to give her air.

When I came up to the surface several seconds later I realized that I hadn't been sufficiently attentive. I had stayed underwater a little too long. The dolphins seemed somehow to have noticed this before I did, perhaps to have sensed some signal I wasn't aware of.

My theory is that the environment around dolphins offers the best conditions imaginable for a baby's development and thereby for the development of the human race as a whole.

What we found can be summarized as follows.

1. Newborns achieve an immediate contact with dolphins, with no preliminaries. They do not react so quickly to any other animal, tame or wild. Seeing this communication spring up, one gets the feeling that the child and the dolphin have "known each other" for quite a while.

Older children also react in this way, but there is reason to believe that the really young ones achieve the closest contact.

2. In the presence of dolphins, both mothers and children lose their fear of water. Even totally unpractised mothers were able, during our experiments, to swim around completely fearlessly in the open sea with their children if dolphins were present.

To achieve this kind of result, even in a safe swimming pool, generally requires hours of hard training. With dolphins present it happened instantly.

3. Water provides perfect conditions for deep, refreshing sleep. Sea water is particularly good. Its chemical and electrical properties are especially beneficial to the baby's development. The dolphins enhance these properties. Children sleep even more soundly and rest more thoroughly, when the large animals are present.

4. The dolphins really look after the children. The communication which exists between dolphins and children seems to be something which adults cannot experience – something deeper than the communication which exists between adults and children.

5. The physical contact between the dolphins and the children was characterized by an extraordinary care on the

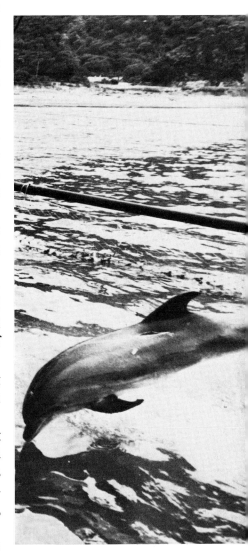

. . . within their humane and gentle social system. Igor believes that dolphins' powerful biofields enable them to sense illness or problems in one another, and even in human beings near them.

123

part of the nine-foot-long animals. They handled the small human beings with a great understanding and purposefulness in their movements, as only an experienced mother can.

'This expedition was only a beginning,' says Igor. 'It is quite probable that continued research in this area can lead to dramatic changes in conditions on earth.

We speak of global conflicts, but opportunities also exist for global contacts between human beings and nature. Up to now, we have for the most part fought against nature by attempting to subjugate and control it. But opportunities also exist for understanding, cooperation and a holistic view of the world.

It seems to me that I often hear this call from the sea, the call for unity and cooperation. Each time I hear of a dolphin saving the life of a human being, it seems it is this call I hear.

Dolphin research has hitherto been characterized by a spirit of aggressiveness and a sense of superiority in a desire to master and control the clever animals. Perhaps what is needed instead is a spirit of cooperation; perhaps we can partake of the dolphins' knowledge and experience. What wisdom the dolphins must have been able to gather during their thousands of years in the seas. They handle our children with tenderness and care. Perhaps our children will be the first to respond in kind. Let them go a step further than we have – let them share the experiences of these gentle inhabitants of the sea.'

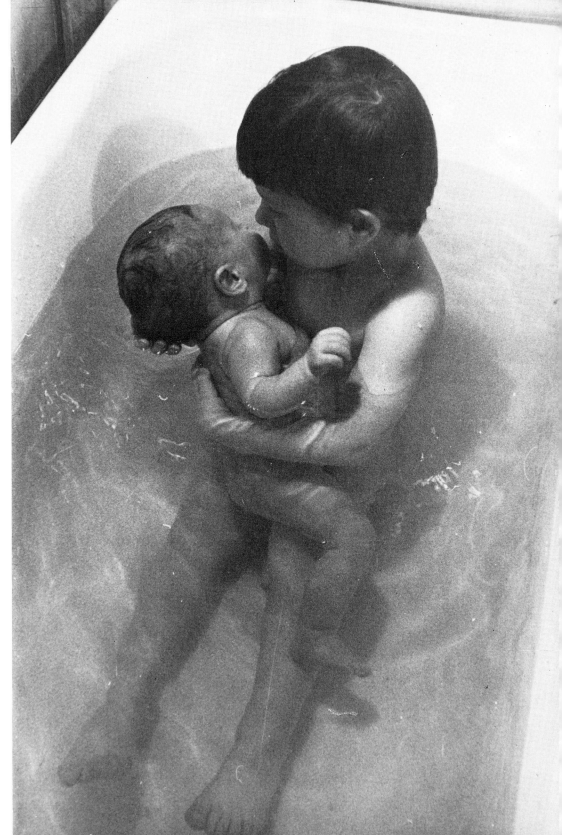

An older sibling can bathe with his new brother or sister, and often becomes an excellent assistant teacher during water-training.

12 How Igor's theories

can be applied to child-raising

Olga and Serge Zjolus are two parents who have, to a certain extent, raised their children according to Igor Tjarkovsky's methods. Here they describe their experiences for us.

'When our son, Nikolai, was born we decided to give him an athletically-orientated upbringing: I was a professional swimmer and my husband taught scuba-diving at a military academy.

In the beginning, unfortunately, we had no ready-made method at hand for stimulating a newborn baby's physical development. When Nikolai was three weeks old, however, we began getting him used to the water. Our first step was training him to hold his breath. We splashed water in his face, gradually began pouring small amounts of water over his head, and finally began dipping him under water.

One can hardly say that he enjoyed this right from the start. He began screaming, and in a way this made things easier. The minute he drew a breath for the next shriek, we dipped his face under water again.

Gradually, Nikolai grew accustomed to these exercises and reacted less violently to them. We came to the conclusion that his screams really didn't mean so much. Screaming is a natural reaction when a child experiences discomfort.

We trained Nikolai to hold his breath by letting him stay underwater for longer and longer periods of time. We began with half a second and gradually worked up to seven to ten seconds, while simultaneously decreasing the length of the intervals between immersions.

By the time Nikolai had learned to hold his breath, he had also learned to dive under the surface of the water on his own. We let him swim around as much as he pleased underwater, near to us. We noticed how important it was to keep a close contact with him. When one of us was nearby the water seemed to hold no threat whatsoever.

When summer came we all went swimming together in a lake. Nikolai sat clinging to one of our backs, his arms wrapped tightly around our necks, and accompanied us on long swims. He thought it was great fun when we dived down and swam a few strokes underwater.

After Nikolai had learned to walk, he was allowed to accompany his father to the sports ground where he worked out. There he was able to do physical exercises, run a couple of laps around the field and try out most of what Serge was doing.

We had also set up some athletic equipment at home, in one corner of the apartment. The two-and-one-half square yards it took up was a space well-used. Not only did the children gain in strength, health and flexibility, it also became their favourite playing-spot. We also immediately noticed the effect upon Nikolai's development.

When he was two years old, he could run a mile and a half, apparently without tiring. At two and a half, he could do exercises on rings and climb to the ceiling on a rope ladder. Even if he grew tired he insisted on climbing down all by himself. Neither of us was allowed to help him. We ourselves believed that it was important for him to learn to handle difficult situations on his own. In this way children learn to be both prudent and inventive.

We are careful to encourage our children when they master new exercises. We pay close attention to what they are doing and when they master something new, we praise them or applaud. This is especially important when the child overcomes his *fear* of something new – it gives him a sense of self-confidence.

One day, some good friends came to visit us with their children. Nikolai started showing the children what he could do on the equipment. While he was hanging way up by the ceiling on a little rope ladder, his five-year-old guest – twice as old as he – began sobbing with fear. When Nikolai came down, the little boy asked, astonished – "Weren't you afraid up there?" Nikolai didn't even answer him. He just started playing with something else. We realized that he didn't understand what the boy meant.

When Nikolai, at the age of three, went to a gym with his eighteen-month-old sister Nadia, both children immediately felt at home there. Nikolai immediately began doing somersaults on a mat, then went on to more complicated vaults and tried out the all-purpose gymnastic apparatus. Nadia preferred the wall bars and the trampoline.

The children's greatest source of delight, however, was the water. Nikolai could lie floating in the water (on his back) when he was five months old, Nadia when she was four months old. At the age of fifteen months Nikolai began diving underwater, and when Nadia was a year old she could swim several metres underwater.

If Nadia made more rapid progress than Nikolai, this was because her parents were more experienced and because Nikolai became a sort of "assistant teacher" for his little sister.

The whole family then began going to a marvellous swimming pool. Nikolai, then two years and five months old, soon felt at home there. He dived and splashed around like a little seal. He especially enjoyed jumping into the water from the starting blocks. Once he had jumped in he was in no hurry to come up to the surface again, he swam in every direction under the water. After a while, Serge and Nikolai climbed up to the three-metre board. The minute his father suggested that they jump from it, Nikolai was off. Serge didn't even have a chance to see him jump.

After this Nikolai jumped off the high-dive by himself over and over again, equally delighted each time.

It wasn't difficult to persuade him to try jumping off the five-metre board. He climbed up all by himself, walked up to the edge, squatted and . . . although we had expected him to jump, we couldn't help catching our breaths when the little fellow (he wasn't even two and a half yet) kicked off from the edge and fell, slowly, slowly it seemed, down towards the water. When he came up he swam over to the ladder and shouted, "Daddy, I flew! Like a bird!"

He jumped many times after that, but we'll never forget that very first time.

It took Nikolai two months to learn to dive with a scuba unit: by then it was time for the whole family to take a trip to the ocean. The weather was fantastic when we arrived – the sea was calm, the water clear and warm. Nikolai put on his diving fins, went down to the beach and swam fearlessly out into the water. When he returned from this first encounter with the sea, he only asked, "Why doesn't this water taste good?"

When he put on his scuba gear and together with his father dived down to the sea-bottom, he was beside himself with wonder and fascination. All around him fish were swimming and crabs were crawling, and the rocks were covered with algae and sea-anemones. It was all so interesting that his eyes nearly popped out of his head. One moment he was chasing a starfish, the next picking up as many shells as he could hold.

Serge and Nikolai were having so much fun on the bottom of the sea that they completely forgot about the time.

130

Suddenly, Serge noticed that Nikolai had stopped playing and had begun swimming up to the surface. When he came up he complained that the "air was bad" in his tank. In actual fact it had run out.

It's difficult to keep track of the time underwater without a watch, when there are so many interesting things to look at. After this incident we grew more careful. We came to the conclusion that a half-gallon tank of compressed air will last a two-and-a-half-year-old child twelve to fifteen minutes.

During this visit to the sea, Nikolai had the opportunity to meet some dolphins. Along with his father, he was allowed into their underwater enclosure. He was also allowed to feed them fish from his hand. The dolphins approached him cautiously, snapped the fish out of his hand and swam away again. The doubt and uncertainty which the child and the animals displayed towards each other in the very beginning was soon replaced by mutual sympathy.

The dolphins also proved to be more interested in Nikolai than in adults. They had recently been filmed for television and many people had come into their enclosure. This terrified them so much that even when their trainer came into the water to feed them, they would swim as far away as they could in the opposite direction. They seemed quite simply to have become afraid of people.

But then Nikolai was allowed to visit them. He swam right into the middle of their enclosure with a fish in his hand, and the nine-foot-long creatures swam up to the boy, took the fish out of his hand and began swimming around him. Contact had been established once again: the dolphins clearly sensed the child's trusting and open attitude towards them.

At times during the day, Nikolai and Nadia would go swimming together. Nadia, then sixteen months old, soon became friends with the sea. She loved playing down by the beach, but also enjoyed accompanying Nikolai on long swims. She'd lie floating on her back in the water and

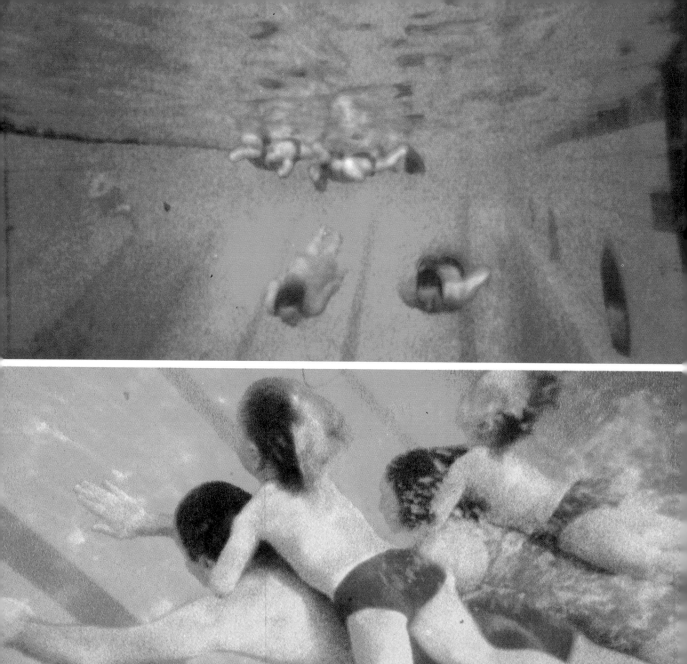
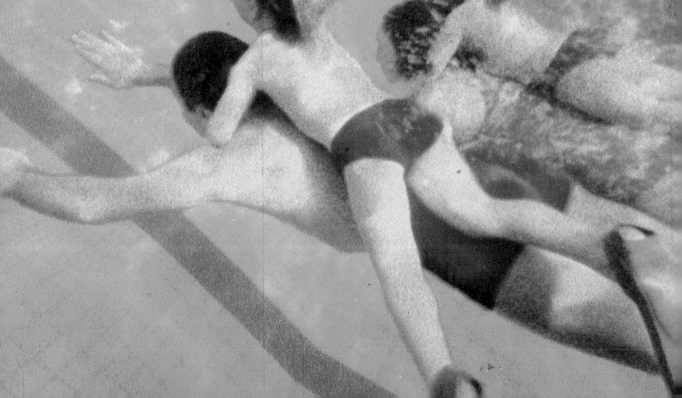

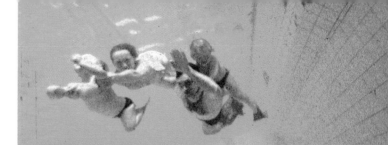

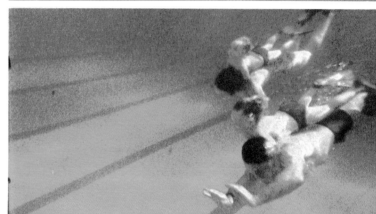

The entire Ziolus family loves to swim and dive. In these photographs, we see them swimming together across the pool. Sometimes Nikolai and Nadia swim by themselves, using fins to get up speed. At other times they hitch a ride on the parents' backs, either underwater or on the surface.

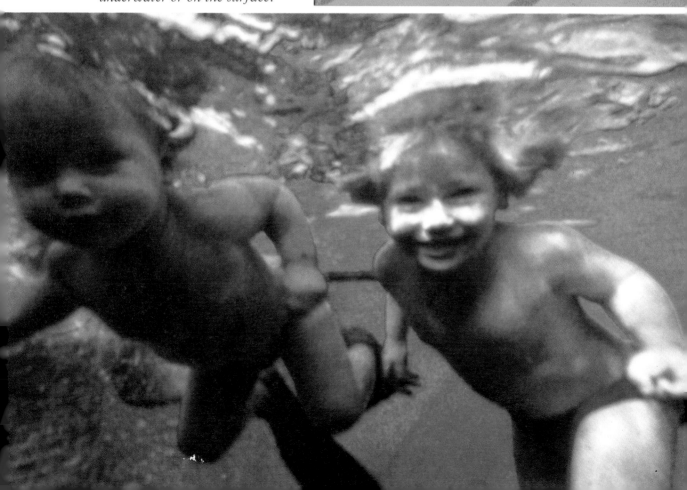

Nikolai would tow her out ten or twenty yards from the shore. While he dived down to the bottom, she lay floating on the surface, mostly on her back. Sometimes she turned over on her stomach and swam a few strokes, then rested on her back again. When Nikolai had finished diving he would tow her back to the shore, and they'd both lie in the sun and dry off.

One day when the waves were high, Olga and Nikolai swam 150 yards out from the shore to play. Nikolai had an inflatable rubber tube around him. They played in the waves for half an hour, and then it was time to swim back. By then the wind had changed, however, and it was now blowing out from the shore. It was blowing so hard that there were white caps on the water and they found themselves being carried out to sea.

Olga told Nikolai that he'd have to swim to the shore by himself because she couldn't tow him. He gave her his rubber tube and started swimming in to shore. It was tough going, and now and then he turned on his back to rest, although he continued paddling even then.

It took them nearly an hour to reach the shore.

We had a wonderful time by the sea with the children. All too soon, it was time to return to Moscow. Once home, we immediately continued our training in a swimming pool.

When Nadia was twenty months old, she could swim 500 yards at a stretch. We also began taking the children with us to a sports ground where they could run, jump, climb and try out different types of gymnastic apparatus. They were already familiar with several from our "athletic corner" at home. The children watched what the athletes were doing with interest and took note of the exercises which we ourselves did.

During the autumn we went to the pool two or three times a week, and at home there was daily exercise and practice on the equipment.

It was also time for Nikolai and Nadia to begin attending

the day-care centre. The three-year-old Nikolai and the one-and-a-half-year-old Nadia were the youngest in their groups, but they handled the adjustment period without problem and participated with great zest in the other children's activities.

One day, at the pool, a young mother came over to us and asked if it was too late to begin training her child to swim – he was now one and a half years old. If not, how should she begin?

We are convinced that it is never too late. The earlier one begins, however, the better it is for the child and the parents.'

13   Water-training for all

'Igor, you say that water has such fantastic properties. It decreases the organism's energy consumption and facilitates the transmission of bio-energy. Can't all this enormous potential for development be put to practical use in other fields?'

'Yes, I'm sure it can. I have no technical knowledge in areas other than my own, but I'm sure that other specialists who examine my results will be able to come up with many answers to these questions.

An agronomist, for example. I'm certain that water-training could be useful in animal-raising. Raising pigs in water should make them grow larger and develop faster. But as I said, I know too little about agriculture to say exactly how my findings could be applied. I know more about medicine, and I have several ideas in this field. Adults could be treated in water in the same way that I've treated premature and handicapped newborns. Operations could even be carried out in water.

I'll tell you about an experiment which I honestly hadn't planned. One day I accidentally dropped a box full of newborn baby animals on to the floor. They apparently received serious injuries, many of them appeared half-dead. Well, I let half of the baby animals stay in the box, and carefully tilted the others over into a basin of water. The animals allowed to lie in the water survived, and the others died. The reason for this, of course, is that weightlessness in water reduces oxygen and energy requirements so that the body's resources can to a greater extent be used to repair injuries.

This knowledge could be put to use in medical treatment. Just think: if someone has a serious accident, what do we do? First we carry him on a shaky stretcher, then jolt him off to the hospital in an ambulance. His injuries only increase. Instead, the injured person could be transported in a tub of water, or in a flexible water-bag if this is more practical. The details can always be discussed: the tub's form; whether the injured person should be supported so that his face remains above water or whether he should wear an oxygen mask, and so on. The important thing is to make the fullest possible use of water's ability to support and protect the body and decrease oxygen consumption.

Transportation and treatment in water could also be of great significance to patients with serious diseases of respiratory and circulatory systems – heart and lung problems, infarcts and so on.

Oxygen supply is also a problem during certain major operations. One solution could certainly be "hydro-surgery", operations in or under water, and there are various possibilities here. One is to raise the area to be operated upon above the surface of the water while keeping the rest of the body immersed. Another is to immerse the entire body in water, and carry out the operation underwater as well.

The water or liquid being used must naturally be sterilized to avoid infection. During our underwater births, however, this has not proved to be a problem.

Can one see sufficiently to operate underwater, especially

if the water mixes with blood? This could present a problem, but a flowing stream of water which is constantly being replaced might be one solution. This in itself would be one advantage of hydrosurgery over conventional surgery, in which the wound always gets more or less besmeared however much one cleans it off and ties off veins. Anyone who has ever cut himself on a shell while swimming in the ocean knows how clearly visible the wound is through the water, and how the blood is continuously washed away.

Another advantage of hydrosurgery is that in water, the organ being operated on does not collapse and become deformed, but can maintain its volume.

Naturally, I realize that hydrosurgery will pose many problems during its developmental phase. But these problems are no more complicated than a thousand others which medical technology has already solved. I am convinced that hydrosurgery will be of great value to us in the future.

One example of how problems can be solved is the fact that we – both in the Soviet Union and in other countries – are already delivering babies underwater. This was completely unthinkable not so long ago!'

14

A key

to the future

'During the last few decades, the earth's inhabitants have been increasingly confronted with questions about future development,' says Igor.

'In the past, prophets who made dark predictions about the future were dismissed as mentally disordered. Today, more and more people are viewing the future with pessimism. We have realized that the future of the world is something which concerns us all, something which we cannot put aside until some vague tomorrow or simply leave to those in power.

All our energies are needed to solve the complex problems now facing humankind. But can we gather together *greater* energies? This is the question to which I have devoted the last twenty years of my life.

Anthropologists say that the development of the human brain has been at a standstill for many thousands of years. Just consider the possibilities which would open up for every one of us if the brain's potential were to be increased; if future generations had a greater ability to solve difficult problems.

I often speak of an "evolutionary impasse". I am

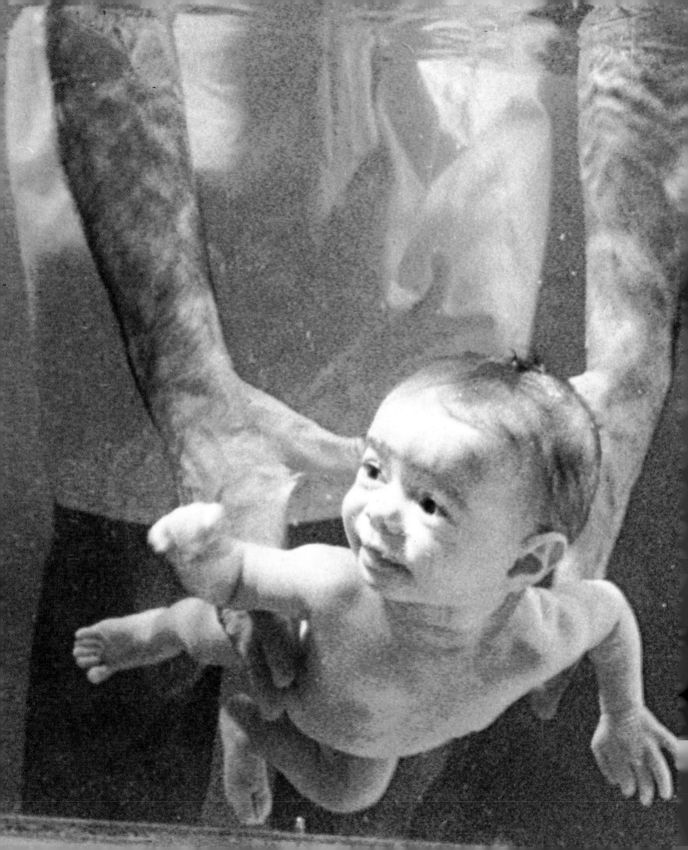

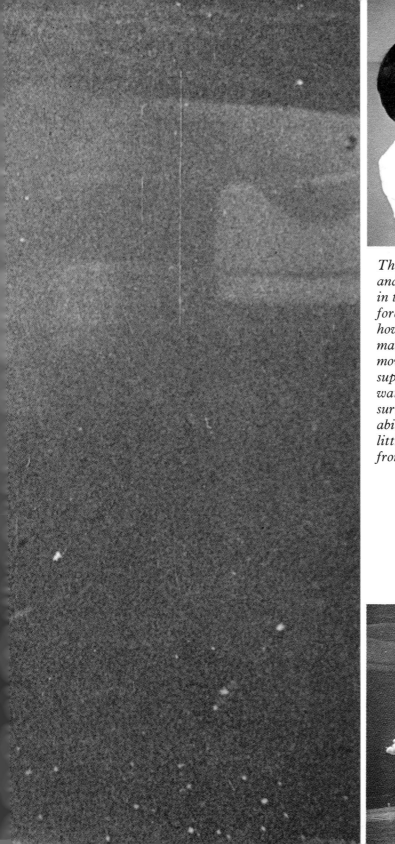

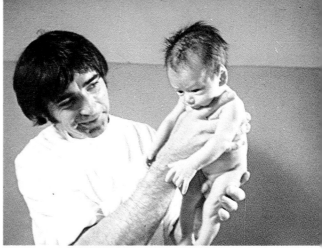

The newborn child, so helpless and unsteady when it is held in the air and exposed to the force of gravity. In water, however, it has full mobility, makes precise, purposeful movements and doesn't need support for its head. In the water, it can investigate its surroundings and try out its abilities – all it needs is a little caress, a little guidance from an adult's hand.

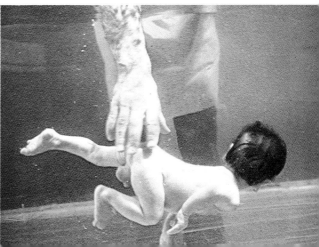

referring to the grim fact that land-animals' way of giving birth, a brusque step from an existence in the waters of the womb to a life subject to the force of gravity, sets definite limits upon the brain's capacity.

Only the strongest and crudest brain functions survive the trauma of birth. The most sensitive and valuable ones collapse. When the organism's resources immediately following birth are insufficient and the body must economize, it does so by drawing on the brain – on its capacity and potential for development. It sounds absurd, but it's true.

Under these circumstances, can there be talk of our having potential for development?

This is the area on which I have concentrated in my research. I've tried to point out ways in which we can get around this impasse. My solutions, however, cannot be encompassed within the bounds of conventional thinking or the limits of conventional disciplines. A new way of thinking is needed, and this is easier said than done.

In the beginning, I too had great difficulty in accepting facts which didn't fit into the picture of the world which I, like everyone else, had been brought up with. I often had to restrain myself from rejecting objective, calculated results. I didn't *want* to accept them, for they conflicted not only with present scientific attitudes but also with what is referred to as "common sense". It was only with great difficulty that I came to realize that "common sense" is often no more than a collective delusion and that we, in this period of global problems and sophisticated technology, have a tendency to disregard simple and very obvious truths.

We have, for example, totally ruled out the possibility of human beings adapting to a life in water. This is regarded as an axiom. No scientist has ever bothered to investigate whether it really is impossible. Because this axiom exists, scientists do not *want* to take notice of the thousands of facts which clearly demonstrate that adaptation to water is not only possible but also essential to the development of our physical and intellectual potential.

I have reports and figures from our experiments with animals which clearly demonstrate how life in water makes animals healthier, stronger, more intelligent and longer-lived. The effects on human beings are the same, though one can never directly translate results of animal experimentation to people. I have not had the opportunity to conduct equally exhaustive studies of the waterbabies.

I haven't really felt it to be necessary, either. I have looked upon my work as a kind of voyage of discovery or mountain climb. The first time around, one scales a mountain to prove that it's possible. The second time up one can begin studying the details.

People have wondered what these waterbabies will be like when they're grown up. Will their parents feel strange towards them? Will these children have access to feelings and insights which are out of reach for the rest of us?

All of this is possible. The waterbabies have been given a better start in life than the rest of us. Perhaps they know and understand things which we can not comprehend, and which they cannot yet explain to us. They are probably a step ahead of us right from the start, and we'll never be able to close this gap.

As far as my own daughter Veta is concerned, she displays an independence which I trace to her early life in water. She is accustomed to doing as she pleases, and has difficulty submitting to rules and regulations. When she began swimming for a coach, she could not psychologically tolerate the monotony. After following instructions for fifteen minutes, she grew bored. It is only with great effort that she can sit through a forty-five minute lecture, and she is not prepared to adjust to her companions simply to keep the peace.

Independence and initiative were also qualities found in French studies of the Leboyer children's development. In

Cologne, West Germany, researchers have studied four- to six-year-olds who began swimming at an early age and compared them with a control group.

The swimmers developed much more rapidly than the non-swimmers. Researchers are now discussing what the direct causes of this can be. Whatever they are, it is evident that the swimming-children, though only trained for an hour each week, display greater independence and ability to handle new situations, better concentration and precision and higher intelligence. Their motor and social skills were also superior to those of their peers.

My colleagues and I also consider the waterbabies to have strong paranormal abilities. They have aptitudes for clairvoyance, telepathy and telekinesis,' says Igor. 'There's nothing strange about it, really, if one assumes that such abilities belong to that group of sensitive brain-functions which are destroyed at birth.

"Have you proved that they have these abilities?" demand my adversaries. My response is that the traditional sciences have barely been able to prove that such abilities exist at all, even in adults. This says more, however, about the state of the sciences than about parapsychology. We have quite simply not yet discovered the methods and techniques needed to measure this aspect of human development.'

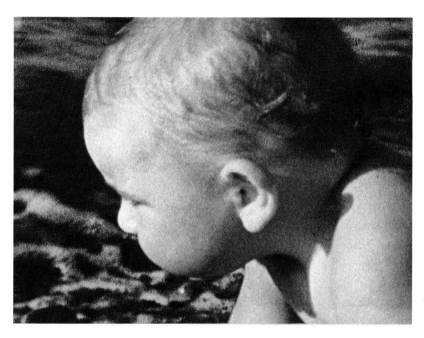

Igor Tjarkovsky believes that a water-trained child has been given a better start in life than the rest of us. And a better start means a better future.

15   Three Swedish voices

on Igor Tjarkovsky

Kent Åke Henricson, paediatrician

Kent Åke Henricson is an assistant physician at a children's clinic in Halmstad, Sweden. Childbirth, from a gynaecological point of view, is not his speciality, but he works with children of all ages, from newborns upwards.

'No one who meets Igor Tjarkovsky can fail to be affected by the enthusiasm he feels for his work, and the sense of calm and confidence he radiates. I consider it a privilege to have been able to meet him and become acquainted with his material, and to have seen him water-train and do acrobatic exercises with children.

This is an exciting and stimulating assignment, to present my views on Igor's work in a book written about him. But it's no easy task. What he has to say is fascinating, but most of what I have learned as a Swedish doctor is turned upside down. It's difficult to comment on Igor's work in a way that does him justice, although I have tried to read the material critically.

I am convinced that in many of the ways Igor Tjarkovsky describes it can be beneficial for babies and children to spend time in water, even though I have not had the chance to observe his more advanced water-training.

These children develop more rapidly, have larger, stronger, more solidly-built bodies and are better equipped to handle physical hardships. I had the opportunity to examine a five-month-old child whose fine and gross motor skills (ability to carry out small and large movements) proved to be equal to those of a nine-month-old.

In the West, more and more attention is beginning to be paid to the fact that babies, even from earliest infancy, have a need to move around. At a recent world congress for physical therapists, for example, a physical training programme for children between the ages of four and nine was presented.

I consider Igor to be completely correct in maintaining that it is of great value to newborns to be allowed to turn, dive, lie on their stomachs and use their limbs instead of lying flat on their backs in a basket. This in itself must encourage improved development.

One must bear in mind, however, that Igor Tjarkovsky lives and works in a country where it is much less common for newborns to be allowed to move their bodies freely. In the Soviet Union it is still common practice to swaddle infants, a custom which transforms them into helpless bundles for several months. This brings us to the difficulties involved in judging Igor's work fairly. His point of departure and traditions are not our own.

In the Soviet Union, childbirth and child-care are differently managed and by different standards from the West. This must be remembered when one is judging the risks involved in carrying out an underwater delivery without the highly technological resources we have available to us for control and intervention.

In the Soviet Union, methods and norms for child-rearing (indeed the entire attitude towards children) differ greatly from ours. In Igor's discussion of the "waterpeople" of the future who will be mentally, physically and spiritually superior to today's adults, one recognizes features of an "übermensch" (superman) attitude. It is an elitist way of thinking which is alien to us in the West.

Last but not least, the entire scientific tradition in the Soviet Union is different from our own. In the West, scientific work follows certain rules. Researchers first describe their methods and materials. They then give an account of their results, which are then discussed before the summary is presented. While the research is underway, work-in-progress reports are also published. For scientific work to be accepted, it must be accounted for so precisely that others will be able to repeat the experiments and produce the same results.

We never receive such accounts from the Soviet Union. For this reason it is difficult to compare their findings with our own. Igor's account of his many years of work is, from our point of view, quite inadequate.

It's a pity his results are not better supported, especially since we have very little to compare them with. Incidentally, many of the experiments he has done with children would be judged unethical and unfeasible by Swedish doctors.

To sum up, it is difficult to know what to accept and what to reject of the material Igor presents here. We know that some of his statements are incorrect; for example, his statement about the oxygen requirements of newborns. In other contexts his wording is incorrect. He speaks for example of "premature" babies, where this is a broad concept which covers several different types of developmental disturbances.

Igor Tjarkovsky probably has an inadequate background in biology, or rather, an education which emphasizes different areas of knowledge from our own. These are factors which often make it difficult to credit what he presents. No sooner has one caught him in an error, however, than he comes up with a statement which leaves one uncertain. It is impossible to say whether or not it is correct. The human body and its functions have not yet been completely understood; new substances and processes are constantly being discovered.

When it comes to the large part of Igor's work dealing with parapsychological thought, I remain sceptical. My background and training do not qualify me to express my opinions on anything other than the training of babies. As regards the other, alleged, positive effects, only the future can provide us with answers – and perhaps the research being carried out in this area in the United States and West Germany, among other countries.

On the other hand, I do not feel that the parapsychological and cosmic dimensions are necessary for an appreciation of Igor's water-training programme. The critical viewpoints I've expressed are in no way intended to minimize the value of Igor Tjarkovsky's unique and original contributions to our knowledge of child development. I am convinced that water-training has positive effects upon children, even though I, like Igor, have been subjected to backbiting when I've asserted this. "What's the point of people being in water? We're land animals, after all . . .", and so on.

Even if I am personally not prepared to treat weak newborns in tanks of water (nor, presumably, is any other Swedish doctor), I must point out that here in Sweden, physical therapists carry out a great deal of their rehabilitation work with older handicapped children in water. Their experiences prove Igor to be entirely right. Water-training can work wonders for feeble and handicapped children – both for their ability to move and for their self-confidence.'

Lars Redvall, gynaecologist

Lars Redvall is assistant senior physician at the women's clinic at Mölndal General Hospital.

'The ideas which Igor Tjarkovsky presents are in many ways fascinating and valuable. Much of his thinking is based upon a cultural background extremely different fron ours, however, which makes it difficult to take a stand.

I sympathize for the most part with Igor Tjarkovsky's attitudes towards delivery. He offers many valuable insights. It is undoubtedly relaxing and comfortable for women to deliver in water, if they are psychologically prepared for it and have a positive attitude towards the idea.

The delivery positions which physicians have recommended from the 19th century and onwards are physiologically absurd and incredibly uncomfortable. It is only the solidly established respect for authority which has induced women to adapt to these rules. There's not much left of all this today, however. Nowadays, women make use of the delivery bed in extremely undogmatic ways. They prop themselves up with pillows in various positions, lie on their stomachs or crouch on all fours. A tub of water would be a conceivable contribution to a modern delivery.

I believe, as Igor Tjarkovsky does, that the risk of infection should not present a problem for underwater delivery, as long as the woman is only exposed to her own bacteria. The situation could be different in a hospital where problems are already developing with the occasional "infection on the loose". Institutionalized, production-line deliveries in water are obviously not to be recommended.

I don't want to give the impression of being a sour-tempered reactionary. Despite my positive interest, however, I'd like to take up a few places in this book where Igor Tjarkovsky presents us with facts which conflict with knowledge I've gained from books or through experience.

153

He spends a great deal of time discussing the changes in cell activity which occur when the body is immersed in water and freed from the force of gravity. On the one hand, these changes do not have a tangible influence upon the inner organs. Pressure conditions in the abdominal cavity and around the brain do not change appreciably because these organs are always suspended in liquid. On the other, neither oxygen nor energy consumption is affected to any great degree when we are weightless, as experiments on astronauts have shown.

Igor's description of how he floated unconscious in the water for hours is also improbable, to say the least. An unconscious person will normally, after a short time, take on a prostrate position in the water – that is to say, will float with the shoulder area upwards and the face under the surface of the water. An unconscious person cannot float in the water and breathe.

Igor's statements regarding the way in which premature infants can, in some cases, endure a lack of oxygen better than fully developed babies are correct. But his figures are not, according to our experience. Newborns cannot endure a lack of oxygen for ten to fifteen minutes. Even after ten minutes, irreparable brain damage has occurred.

As regards his discussion of bio-energy, biofields and healing, I am not aware of any research in the West which provides clear evidence for the truth of his statements. Our experience seems to touch on certain points, however: Igor believes, for example, that maternity hospitals provide an unhealthy environment because the biofields of many tense people intrude upon one another. We, for our part, are aware of the way in which the fear aroused in a woman by an unfamiliar and stressful hospital environment can trigger the release of hormones which disturb certain physiological processes during labour.

To conclude: Igor describes the way in which babies, when swimming, can find their way to their mother in the dark by using their sense of taste. I'd have to see this to believe it, even though it is common knowledge that a newborn baby can recognize its mother by her smell after only a few days, for example when she breast-feeds it.'

Annelie Traugott, child psychologist

A child psychologist working at Danderyd Hospital.

'I became acquainted with Igor Tjarkovsky by chance, in Moscow, and found him a fascinating and exciting person.

Igor Tjarkovsky considers it his mission in life to develop and publicize a method of delivery and a way of handling the newborn child which will minimize the traumatic effects of birth and adjustment to a life outside the mother. The tiny human being can in this way begin its life with full access to its potential for development.

During recent years, much attention has been directed, within the field of psychotherapy, to children's very earliest life experiences. We have, by various means, brought up these early memories to the level of consciousness, and seen them as important pieces of the jigsaw puzzle of human development.

My first meeting with Igor took place in his home. His youngest son Kolja was then a week old. He lay naked on the bed, in itself an unusual sight in the Soviet Union where people generally wrap children up in thick layers of clothing. His parents picked him up and carried him around a lot in a horizontal position, with one hand under his stomach to support his back. They said that this was good for the breathing and for the back muscles.

During my visit, Igor filled the bathtub with water and showed me how he carries out the very earliest water-training. He has a calmness about him, a warm, loving harmony, which at that moment was filling the little bathroom. Freedom from the fear of water, from fear of the training situation, is essential if the experience is to be a positive one for the child.

Little Kolja moved around in the water with calm, relaxed movements. His face, with his clear, wide-open eyes, looked serene and curious under the water. At short intervals his little face popped up out of the water for air. The whole experience affected me deeply.

What is uniquely new about Igor's work, and what really fires the imagination, is the philosophical aspect of his theories on development, which he is working to document scientifically, and which are also presented in this book.

The portion of his work which is perhaps the easiest for this country to accept, however, is the carefully-expressed training programme for parents.

The mother is encouraged to spend as much time as possible in the water and to begin her own water-training as early as possible during her pregnancy. An important part of the mother's training is practice in moving and looking around *underwater*. According to Igor the baby, even as a foetus, learns a great deal which it can later put to practical use. The father is also encouraged to spend time training in the water.

My belief as a psychologist is that this training offers parents increased opportunities for teamwork and interplay around the awaited child. It also helps the mother to focus upon her growing body in a positive and sensual way.

The training programme also includes detailed instruction about the delivery and regular meetings at the pool with parents of newborns (together with their children) as well as other expectant parents. As part of their preparation, the expectant parents are also, if possible, allowed to observe an underwater delivery.

Igor's programme is, in other words, a broadly conceived "education" for parents who plan to deliver and train their child in water. The programme provides an intensive physical, mental, and social preparation for receiving a new life into the world.'